"Unstoppable Attitude"

"Unstoppable Attitude"

✦

Facing the Challenge of Cancer

The Ten Principles of "Unstoppable Attitude" To Achieve Your Goals

PeterMax Miller

iUniverse, Inc.
New York Bloomington Shanghai

"Unstoppable Attitude"
Facing the Challenge of Cancer

iUniverse books may be ordered through booksellers or by contacting:

iUniverse
1663 Liberty Drive
Bloomington, IN 47403
www.iuniverse.com
1-800-Authors (1-800-288-4677)

Because of the dynamic nature of the Internet, any Web addresses or links contained in this book may have changed since publication and may no longer be valid.

ISBN: 978-0-595-49224-4 (pbk)
ISBN: 978-0-595-61014-3 (ebk)

Printed in the United States of America

www.UnstoppableAttitude.com

To all cancer patients, their spouses, partners, and loved ones that have run their "races" before me, particularly to those, that despite their valiant efforts, were not able to cross the "survival finish line" of cancer. You and your very loved and missed cancer heroes are the true champions of this amazing process. It is your hard work, dedication, and ultimate sacrifices that have paved the way for myself and thousands of others to cross the cancer "survival finish line". It is you whom I love, and for you whom the memories of my "first," "second" and "third" Ironman® events are written for.

—PeterMax

Contents

Foreword
by
Carol Zapalowski, M.D., PhD.

"Unstoppable Attitude" is a book that will be appreciated by people from all walks of life. This book is able to put our feelings and fears about cancer into words and helps us to understand and overcome them. You will find yourself absorbed by this book whether you are an elite athlete, a person facing or having beaten cancer, or a loved one of that cancer patient. You will find this book inspirational if you are someone who is looking for the motivation to allow you to attain the next level of whatever you are trying to accomplish. This might be a faster time in your next race, a promotion at work, or a better relationship with a child or parent. If you are a coach trying to come up with new ways to help a trainee gain confidence and win his or her next event (or get that personal record), you will find PeterMax Miller's thoughts and ideas distinctly beneficial. If you are a health care professional, reading about Mr. Miller's unstoppable attitude will bring goose bumps and tears. It will allow you to work through the times during which finding a diagnosis was particularly difficult and frustrating for everyone involved, despite your best efforts. After reading PeterMax's point of view, you will be better prepared the next time you come across this inevitable situation.

PeterMax Miller is truly an amazing human being. His analogy of going through treatment for cancer and training for a race is a unique and inspirational way to view one's journey through cancer therapy. As a member of PeterMax's team, I had the opportunity to personally witness his unstoppable attitude. Like every good athlete, he prepared for the challenge. In his first Ironman® competition, he did not have a clear idea of what lay before him, but he did not allow uncertainty to become a barrier. In fact, it became one of his greatest strengths. Similarly, in the battle of cancer, he frequently was faced with the unknown, and not only the unknowns of surgery, radiation and chemotherapy. He faced the most difficult of unknowns in the world of medicine—the frustrations involved in a diagnosis which is hard to uncover. With his experience from the Ironman® Triathlon, PeterMax managed these obstacles with amazing finesse. His attitudes about cancer, athletic competition, and life in general are truly amazing and humbling.

The only sport I have ever coached is soccer when my children were quite young. PeterMax refers to me as one of his coaches and admittedly, I never would have described myself as such. But being one of PeterMax's coaches in his last two races is something that has and will always inspire me as a physician and perhaps, even more so, in my everyday life. Every coach remembers their best and most committed athletes and that is most certainly true for my encounters with Mr. Miller. As physicians, we learn from our patients' experiences and are then able to better serve our future patients. The ability to be a part of PeterMax's unstoppable attitude just because I am a physician is an experience that I wish for every coach, no matter what the sport or subject.

You don't have to be an elite athlete or a cancer survivor to learn from Peter's stirring account of his experiences. I have been laughed at by some of my more athletic friends for wearing a T-shirt from a local race on which the phrase 'Finishing is Winning' is written on the back. But in some races, and for many of us, finishing IS winning. It is from the hours of preparation that we learn and benefit and gather our strength. Peter's philosophy about how better to prepare oneself for and how to imagine oneself completing that difficult race (or that difficult time in your own life or that of a loved one) is nothing less than awe-inspiring. His infectious attitude is guaranteed to help inspire and guide you through your next personal challenge.

Introduction

Dad,

The coolest thing about becoming an Ironman® is that it is a life-long membership.
You are an Ironman®. You can do this!
Happy Birthday
I Love You

Greg

The above note, from my son Greg, was written in the book *"25 Years of the Ironman® Triathlon World Championship"* he sent, to me, for my fifty-fourth birthday. It was also my first day in the hospital for high dose chemotherapy in preparation for a bone marrow transplant. I was starting my "third" Ironman® event. The first was the "ultimate test of endurance", the swim, bike, and run Ironman® World Championship endurance race on the Big Island of Hawaii. The second one to conquer a bone cancer, and this third one to conquer a recurrence of that cancer. Before walking into the hospital, I already knew I would be a winner. In my mind, I had already beaten cancer. The Bone Marrow transplant process was going to be a "grueling formality."

When I arrived in my hospital room, I was greeted with the same positive message, and birthday balloons tied to the bed, from my daughter, Kelly.

Dad,

Happy birthday!
I know you can do this—I'm proud of you!
Love,

Kel

It is a remarkable thing when your kids provide you the same advice you have given them for years. The "You can do this" message is something I have always told both Greg and Kelly. They are both "can do this" young adults. First, they are accomplished "solid, good citizens" of the world. They are adventurous, applying their "can do this" attitudes to traveling, moving to new places, meeting new people, and learning new things. They are loyal to their friends, and truly respect all good people. Of course, they are accomplished athletes, both are marathoners and triathletes. Greg and Kelly have told me that their "go anywhere," "do anything," "can do this," and "no obstacles" attitude came from me. I cannot take full credit, but I feel it is my greatest accomplishment, and when I think of it, I take a moment to enjoy that satisfying "my world is a perfect place" feeling.

"Unstoppable Attitude"

The most profound event of my life, in terms of a lasting knowledge of how to channel my positive attitude to accomplish "big" things, was training for and completing the World Championship Triathlon on the big island of Hawaii in October, 1982. It was the sixth Ironman® World Championship event, and just the third time it was held in Kona, on the Big Island of Hawaii.

The event was, and still is, much more than a race consisting of 2.4 miles of rough water swimming in the ocean, bicycling 112 miles in the lava fields, and running 26.2 miles into dusk. Two impressions of the event I distinctly remember was seeing extremely healthy people "built like trees," and an instant seemingly "long time" camaraderie with fellow athletes I met and knew for only the four days that I was on the island.

I remember the apprehension I had with the long distance I swam from the safety of the rocky shore line, and seeing the bottom of the ocean some ninety feet below, while swimming towards a turn around boat that I could not see until I was quite close to it.

I remember the wind that always seemed against me while bicycling over the newly black topped Queen Kamehameha Highway that gripped my tires, and the searing heat through black lava fields that made it seemed like I was riding and running through the bottom of a charcoal grill. Most of all, I remember the year of training marked by a consistent improvement in endurance fitness, skills in the three disciplines, and learning my "rules" to maintain a "can do" positive attitude, no matter the degree of difficulty and adversity.

In 1982, there were still a lot of unknowns about the ability to finish the Ironman® World Championship, the "ultimate event" in the world of ultra-endurance. The event is a result of combining three previously existing races together, to be completed in succession: the Waikiki Rough Water Swim (2.4 miles), the Around-Oahu Bike Race (112 miles, which was originally a two-day event) and the Honolulu Marathon (26.2 miles). Training for the event was a "guess"; there were no books on such endurance training. Nutrition along the course, as I remember, consisted of chocolate chip cookies, plenty of water, and bananas. The science of training and nutrition for such an event was quite simple!

In the early 1980's there was an erroneous belief that, if you could run a marathon, you would never die of heart disease. Both of my parents had passed on too many years before, at the ages of forty seven and forty nine, from heart disease. Therefore, completing the Ironman® World Championship would surely erase this potential from my future! This was not the reason I wanted to complete the Ironman® World Championship, just an interesting "side" benefit, at the time.

Finishing the Ironman® event gives one an instant feeling of immortality. What I remember most of the accomplishment was standing on a rock the next morning, just into the ocean enough to feel the cool lapping waves on my "still hot" sore feet. A sense of accomplishment is a wonderful thing, and at that moment, as one of the two hundred healthiest individuals on the globe, "my world was perfect place," and I had two thoughts: *With my healthy diet and love of active endurance sports, I'll never have a heart disease problem and I would never have a serious medical problem like cancer.* I truly had those two thoughts, and as I have said before; at that moment, "my world was a perfect place."

I approached the Ironman® World Championship event and its grueling training with an "unstoppable" positive attitude. Over the years I have periodically slipped away from my positive attitude "skills" that I developed for the Ironman® World Championship. I realize, however, the times I have used these skills, I always accomplished my goals and reached that fleeting "my world is perfect place" wonderful feeling. As my son wrote and confirmed in the *"25 Years of the Ironman® Triathlon World Championship"* book that he sent to me for my birthday, and my first day in the hospital for a bone marrow transplant, I am an Ironman® with a "life-long membership."

Twenty-two years after my completion of the Ironman® World Championship, I have used my positive attitude to conquer and deal with different medical issues, each could be considered an oxymoron to the title "Ironman®." I have an implanted pacemaker and I am a two-time winner over bone cancer (So much for my two thoughts while standing on that rock after the Ironman® World Championship). I deal with osteoporosis. I also have a pretty "nasty" case of osteoarthritis in my neck, due to a pole vaulting accident in high school. Most recently, I have required treatment for a thyroid problem (common in post cancer patients). When I am focused on goals, however, these types of things become minor "distractions."

Despite these "opportunities of medical issues" to learn about and overcome, I am an accomplished (kids respectfully call me "Old Master") snowboarder. I often hike to higher spots on the ski slopes, and I regularly hike up glaciers during the summer to snowboard down. I mountain bike "up" several mountain trails and passes, roller blade, work out in the mornings, and generally exercise somehow everyday of the week. Physical activity is a very important component of my positive attitude.

In business, when I have utilized my skills of positive attitude, I have the same results of accomplishing my athletic goals. I have passed on the principles of positive attitude to my employees, my university students, and my children. When I see them accomplish their goals, particularly when they consciously use any or all of the ten principles, I get that "my world is a perfect place" feeling. What could be better?

So I pass on my principles of positive attitude, along with my Ironman® experiences, in the water, on the road, and in cancer treatment, where I have been able to validate and put these principles to a "real" test.

1

Be Ready For "Unstoppable Attitude"

Principle 1: Be Inspired

Dorothy and Max, my parents, were very inspiring people. Children are inspired so much while they are growing up, even through their "inspiration resistant" teenage years. You just can't help being inspired by good people. Had my parents lived beyond their final ages of forty-nine and forty-seven, and not had unrelated heart disease, I would have benefited, even more, from their inspiration through my "more open to inspiration" young adult years.

As a child, however, I was extremely open to my Dad's inspiration from his success in business, and his extreme "healthy" attitude towards physical well-being. In business, he was an authentic leader, one that put his own well being and comfort in second place, after his friends and employees. I remember every evening when he came home and emptied his pockets; the one consistent article was a dark blue marble that he always carried throughout his work day. On it was inscribed "the golden rule"—*Do On to Others as You Would Have Others Do On To You.*

The other inspiration I was open to, from my Dad, was his continuous consciousness to be an athlete. This was before the days of popular marathons, local charity runs, and the many small town 10K running races that exist today. This was well before health clubs were available on every corner, not to mention all of the chrome plated exercise machines that now exist for specialized workouts.

This was even before every one knew about "Nike®" running shoes! The New York marathon was a "four lap" event of fewer than one hundred athletes who sipped a very small amount of water (for fear of side aches) and wore hi-top heavily built leather shoes. Healthy activity was, truly, a component of my dad's "unstoppable attitude."

My dad's brother, Freddie, died from Hodgkin's disease at the age of 27 (long before I was born). While he was in college, however, he wrote a paper that analyzed himself, as he would analyze a chemical (he was a chemical engineering student). I remember reading a copy of his paper that circulated among the family, and how in it, he described growing up with my dad. He wrote "I always wanted to be like Max, he was always so athletic and active. In fact, he would wear out three or four pair of shoes, to one pair of mine." Freddie recognized, at a young age, his physical limitations long before he was diagnosed. He too, was inspired by my dad, and wanted to be a coach, in addition to teaching chemistry.

My openness to inspiration from my dad began in the early 1950s. You have to realize that cigarettes where very common, whole milk and red meat were considered the basis of a healthy diet, and "chubbiness" was a sign of a healthy child. During this time, I was having a bit of difficulty with my basic school work. Whether or not this was a form of what we now call "attention deficit disorder" or a stronger distraction attributed to my interest in sports at that time, does not matter. My Dad's solution to help me was to channel my sports interest into an educational experience. He invested in a set of weights, and proceeded to coach me. I remember learning my multiplication tables while "pumping iron." Each math exercise repetition was accompanied by a lift of the barbell! To this day, when I calculate numbers in my head, my arms tend to "curl" an invisible barbell!

Also, early before school, in my Jr. and Sr. high school years I would accompany my Dad for four laps around the "course" in our neighborhood, long before any neighbors were thinking of exercise and long before there was such a thing as "Gatorade!" My dad just knew of his connection between being physically fit, and having a great positive attitude. He constantly passed it on, knowingly or unknowingly to his children.

When I first saw the Ironman® World Championship Triathlon on television, in 1980, I was absolutely amazed! My first thought was basically a "why me?" type of thought. How could I ever do something like that? I thought there were too many obstacles to beat—so I deprived myself of entering and participating in this amazing event the next year. I was, however, open to be inspired by the Ironman® World Championship, and I started running 10Ks and training for marathons. I was not yet thinking of entering, but I was becoming more of an endurance runner. I already had a small amount of bicycle racing experience, mostly local criterium races and a few 100 mile time trials. I learned a lot from these two sports, mainly that I could not always "muscle" my way through a long distance event.—I needed to use my brain for training—a positive attitude and a lot of mental discipline.

I actually learned this the hard way. My second marathon was the New York Marathon in 1981. While I finished in record time for me, I do not remember the finish—I "hit the wall," or completely ran out of energy. I had not used my brain for training, in fact, I under trained, because I was still healing a broken foot from my first marathon in which, ironically, I over trained. I took on a new strategy for my athletic life. No longer was I going to completely exhaust myself at the event or be injured by over or under training. I was going to use my brain to learn all I could about discipline, attitude, training, nutrition, and seek proper coaching.

Once again, I happened to see the Ironman® on television, and this time I surprised myself, as my first thought was *why not me—I can do that!* I was so inspired by those athletes that "showed up!" My next event, the Ironman®, was going to be like a graduation—I was going to learn all I could, train properly and pass my "tests" with achievement or "milestone" goals. The actual race was going to be a celebration of achieving my training goals. I was even quoted in the local newspaper (sports section) with that analogy! The race itself was not a "succeed or fail" event, it was a celebration!

My next step was to look at all the "obstacles" I thought stood in my way. I was going to surpass these obstacles to achieve my goal of finishing the 2.4 mile ocean swim, 112 mile bike race, and 26.2 mile marathon, that comprised the Ironman® World Championship event, in the top third, enjoy the event, and feel good afterwards. One of these obstacles was a bit major—I could "sort" of swim, but not for any distance and my swimming technique, as my swimming coach, Robin, said when he first saw me, was "not a pretty thing to see."

Another obstacle was a worsening arthritic neck, from the pole vaulting accident in high school. While it was an accident that I was fortunate to walk away from, I had to have a portion of my right clavicle removed. Now, at the start of training for the Ironman® World Championship, I realized I had significant pain while running, trouble cycling in an aerodynamic position, and a limited ability to turn my neck to the right, which meant swimming with breathing and vision limited to only my left side. A check with a sports medicine physician, just as I started training for the Ironman® World Championship in October, 1981, revealed that I had actually broken a vertebrae in that 1968 accident, which had now developed into a case of severe arthritis that had spread to several neck vertebrae. At the time, he said I had a "one hundred year old neck" in a 31 year old body.

These kinds of obstacles started to add up, but my desire to compete in the Ironman® World Championship was so strong that I kept focusing on a picture of myself, at the finish line, having accomplished my goals. I was somewhat amused by all of the obstacles I was adding up, yet mentally I was spending more and more of my "thought time" at the finish line, and less and less time thinking of "obstacles."

That's when I realized how we, as humans tend to spend so much thought and time dwelling on the *obstacles* to accomplishing our goals, and so little thought time on the actual *accomplishment* of our goals. I kept picturing myself at the finish line, and finally I started thinking that all of us can make a conscious choice to *"accomplish our goals before we achieve them."* Before I knew it, I was learning the principles of an "unstoppable positive attitude."

Principle 2: Mentally Place Yourself At The Finish Line

And that's what I did—I pictured myself after the race, feeling good, having a good time, cheering on the two thirds of the people finishing behind me.

I want to be very clear; I pictured myself at the finish line—*twelve months before I started the Ironman© World Championship!* I then turned around to look at all the "stepping stones" I used to achieve my goal. These "stepping stones" were once obstacles. What's the difference? Obstacles waste energy that is required to overcome or go around. You have to fight to get over or around obstacles. "Stepping stones," on the other hand, are the easy way to get somewhere. You work with "stepping stones" to accomplish goals, not against. The most amazing thing is that it is our choice to decide something is an obstacle or a "stepping stone."

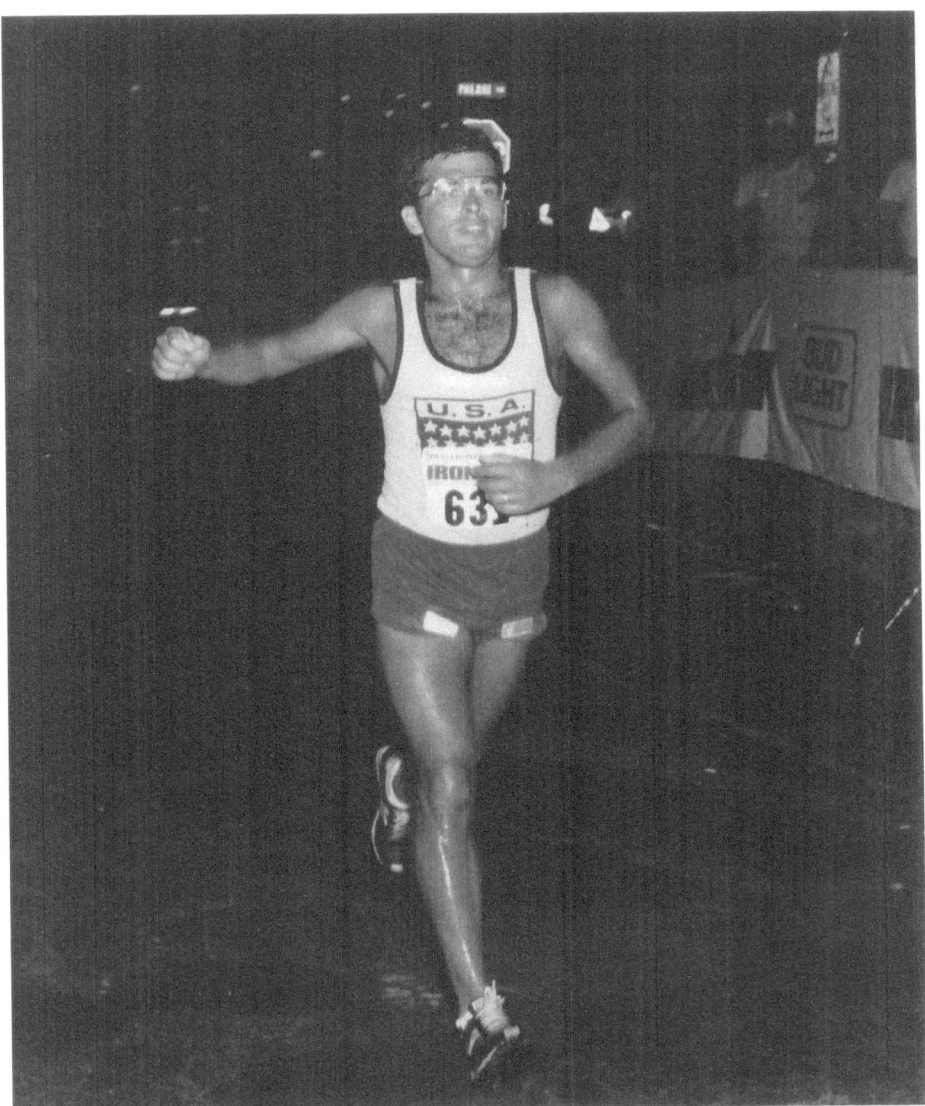

The 1982 Kona Ironman® World Championship Triathlon Finish

Even learning how to swim was no longer an obstacle to be concerned about—it became an opportunity to learn a new fitness skill—it was a "stepping stone" towards my goal. Even training for the first 6 months of the year without being officially qualified and accepted into the race was not an obstacle—in my mind, there was no way this was not going to happen—only the picture of accomplishing my goals. I bought into this thinking so well—You might think I am just able to fool myself easily.

I remember someone asking me, after I had trained so hard for six months—*"so what bib number did you get for the race?"* I replied, *"Oh—I haven't received that yet, they send out the numbers when you are accepted into the race."* He was so shocked—*"how can you train like that for six months without knowing for sure you will be in the race."* I was just as shocked why he would question that—how could he raise that as a doubt? In my mind, I had already run the Ironman© World Championship and accomplished my goals. This was a "done deal!"

During that year I also worked full time. I was responsible for a very important and successful pharmaceutical product launch for a major pharmaceutical company, and I trained for the Ironman© World Championship. My training was an early morning, evening, and weekend adventure. Just to illustrate how times have changed, I was once called into a meeting with the VP of Human Resources to receive a "grilling" about the desired image of the company's executives. Training for the Ironman® World Championship was not the image I should have been portraying, according to that VP. As he said; *"You should not be seen bicycling or running to work, that's what cars are for, and that's why we provide parking."* He went on, *"You should be playing golf as most of our other executives do. That is the kind of image we want around here."* Thank goodness times have changed as many companies, including the company I worked for, encourage a healthy level of physical fitness. I should mention, also, that I recently added a few rounds of golf every year as part of my list of fitness activities that I enjoy!

I enlisted many people to help—my family, a great swim and weight training coach, Robin (who had trained under the legendary swim coach, Doc Councilman), and many positive people who were interested, supportive, and enthused about my goals. I began to notice a "cycle of inspiration." While they thought I was inspiring, I was continuously being inspired by them. There always seemed to be a growing amount of inspiration. One of my "older" friends was my favorite attitude "coach" and would always ask me how many miles I ran or cycled that morning before work. When I gave him the distance—he would always say, regardless of my mileage, *"That's great, PeterMax,"* Then with piercing, but coaching eyes he would drawl out *"but how many were quality miles?"*—A favorite measurement I continue to use for many things, even today, in physical activity, relationships, business, and assignments for my University of Colorado students—*"I want you to write three paragraphs—make that three quality paragraphs."*

In the peak of training, a typical week consisted of over thirty hours of training and looked like this: Bicycle five miles to the fitness club for *serious* swimming and/or weight training at 4:30am with Coach Robin and the local Jr. Olympic swim team. Bicycle another five miles to work, shower and be in the office at 8:00am.

After work, at 5:15pm, I begin a sixty to eighty mile bicycle ride, with Dennis, another inspiring friend and cycling training partner, then I ran a few miles until 7:30pm. Lights were out by 8:30pm. On Saturdays, I usually swam 3 miles, first thing in the morning, and cycled up to 100 miles. Somewhere in each day, I consumed 6,000 to 8,000 calories. In my twelve months of training, I had lifted tons of weights, and covered more than 7,500 miles by land and water.

The event was interesting, to say the least, for the 900 entrants. The 2.4 mile swim was in 3-4ft swells. At the time, I lived in Evansville, Indiana, and despite Indiana not being the ideal place for ocean training (obviously), I finished 50th in the swim. Again, I repeat, enlisting the help of a great swim and weight coach was critical. During the bicycle and run portions of the race, high crosswinds were continuous and the ground temperature reached 117F degrees. During the bicycle portion, I ran into another cyclist, fell and broke, as I later found out, a small piece of my elbow. However, in the race, I was quickly up and back on the bike without being aware of any injury.

When I started the run portion, I discovered I had a pulled muscle, which made it difficult to lift my left leg to run. Those injuries made little difference, as I already completed the event in my mind. I had accomplished my goals before I achieved them! The finish was not a surprise to me. It was a celebration of achieving my goals. What stands out is how completely invincible I felt! I was one of the one thousand or so people in the world that could claim to be an Ironman® World Champion!

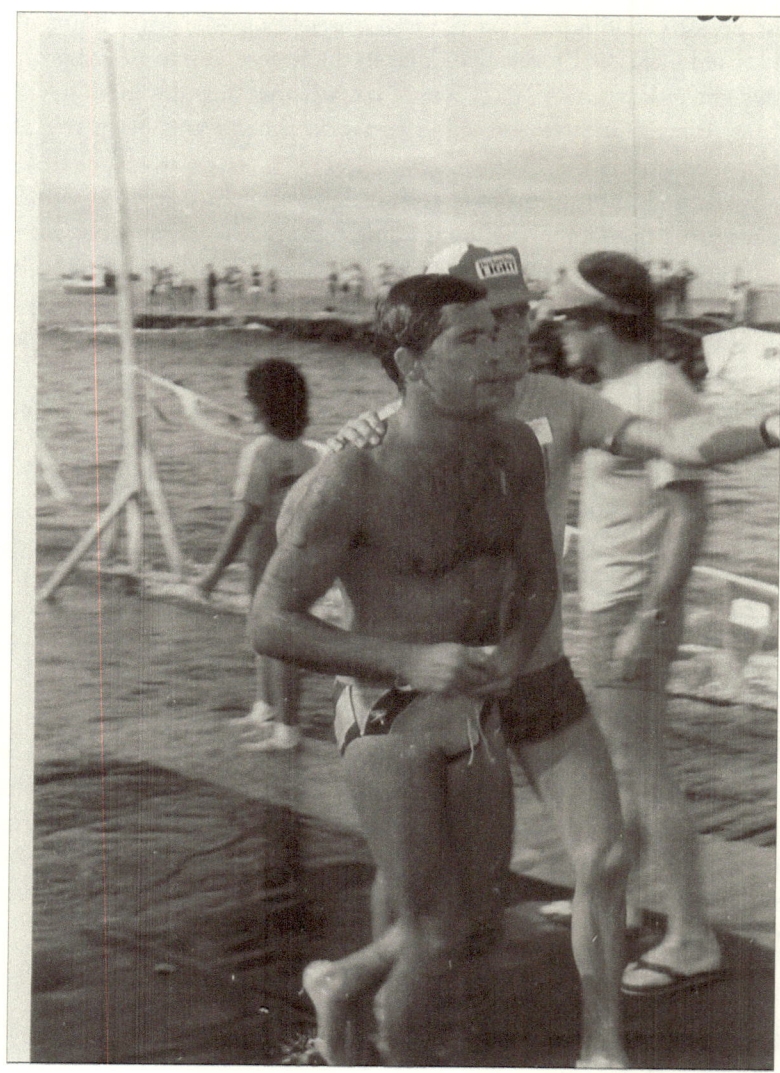

Finishing the 2.4 mile rough water swim in Kona

Principle 3: Live Healthy, Exercise, Eat Well

Since that time, even twenty some odd years ago, I have stayed active at a lesser pace but still at "Ironman® World Championship" quality. Until recent years, I would annually complete several one hundred mile bike rides, well under six hours. I would mountain bike literally "up" the mountain bike trails at Winter Park and Keystone, Colorado, and over several mountain passes. In the spring and summer seasons, I developed a passion for snowshoeing up glaciers to snowboard down. My idea of in-line skating was usually a forty mile "jaunt" with a quick rest stop in the middle of the route to rotate the wheels to maximize "wheel wear."

2

The Beginning Of A New Ironman© Journey

<u>Time Line</u>: 2001: February

In February, 2001, I started getting a pain in my right hip after my Saturdays of snowboarding. My solution, of course, was to return to the mountain on Sundays and "muscle" my way through the pain, ease up during the work week, and "hit" the slopes hard the next weekend. I noticed the worsening of the hip, however, and I was losing turning ability, and experiencing an ever growing amount of pain. I perceived this was something I was not "muscling" my way through and I decided to begin journaling what was going on. The first lines I wrote in the journal were:

> *Journal, Journal, Journal. Something I have so frequently thought would be a good thing to do—something I have so often bought a notebook for, but always used it for business notes. Well—I sense I am on a most important journey of health and wellness that may require utilizing my "unstoppable" Ironman® World Championship positive attitude.*

In April, 2001, I attended two medical conventions for my job, first in New Orleans, and then Orlando. I always liked to walk or run and use the hotel exercise facilities available as much as possible when traveling for business. In New Orleans, I was very limited in time, and my hip "got by" with moderate walking, some weights, and the usual amount of convention standing. The Orlando trip, however, was quite different. I had a huge amount of free "weekend" time in Orlando, as I was setting up the company's exhibit booth. It was about a three mile walk, each way, from the hotel to the convention center, and very flat. I probably walked twelve miles the first day, twenty miles the second day, and another twelve miles each of the next four days. The flat terrain walking, plus the usual convention standing really "lit up" my right hip. I had a pretty tough time sitting on the airplane, returning to Colorado, and was surprised with the level of pain I had while driving my car home.

I managed to snowboard the next weekend, with a competitive friend, and discovered I was unable to make my usual "snappy" turns in the moguls due to the pain and, now also, a growing weakness in my hip. The next weekend, I took a chairlift up 'A-Basin', and realized I could not execute any turns at all!. I carefully made a "straight shot" down the slope on the snowboard and officially "called it a season." I drove home and decided I could no longer "muscle my way through" what ever was going on with my hip. I decided to enlist help from my primary care physician.

Time Line: 2001: February, March, April

My primary care physician told me I had "classic sciatica," prescribed some anti-inflammatory pain relievers, and physical therapy. While I was at my primary care physician, I also asked for a referral to my long time orthopedic physician who, over the years, has treated me for my neck problem.

When I saw my orthopedic physician, a week later, we decided to schedule facet blocks in my neck, which are simply cortisone injections carefully placed at the points of each vertebrae. I also mentioned my sore hip, and he assured me that it sounded like "classic sciatica" and that it would disappear, on its own, in six weeks.

On May 19th, 2001, I arrived at a medical imaging facility for my facet blocks. The interventional radiologist explained that the procedure was "not very pleasant," and that he usually performs the procedure on much older patients. He explained that the procedure was basically inserting needles into my neck, going into a CT scan, then back out to re-position the needles. Once, after several trips in and out of the CT scan, the needles were in the correct position, cortisone would be injected directly to the bone "points" in the vertebrae.

The doctor said he did not advise the procedure unless I was having a lot of pain in my neck, and asked about my level of neck pain. My reply was that it was really low since the pain in my right hip was *"making me crazy"* and my neck, therefore, did not seem as irritated as usual, since my right hip problem was the major limitation of my exercising. He looked at my orthopedic's report and decided that he would at least take a CT scan of my neck. After he started the CT scan, he came into the scan room and exclaimed *"your neck looks like hell."* He further told me that I have a neck that looks *"as bad as any arthritic one hundred year old neck."* He recommended I go back to the primary care physician and have him look at my hip because, if I had the same osteoarthitic degenerative process in my hip as I do in my neck—I probably needed a hip replacement.

I was not surprised. After all, I had traveled thousands of miles running, hiking, climbing, bicycling and walking, and it seemed logical that I may have worn out my hip. I returned to my primary care physician for a check up of my hip, and it "checked out A-OK." I was prescribed more anti-inflammatory medication, and more pain medication. I absolutely hate taking these medications, and I took them sparingly. I obtained another referral to my orthopedic, but could not get in until July 19 after his vacation and, coincidently, after mine.

In July, 2001, I was starting to give in and was taking Percocet™, asprin, an anti-inflamatory, and anything else I could think of for pain, but still on a limited basis when I really hurt. I was now getting very stressed, as the second biotech start-up company I was working for was "flaming out" on the launch pad (going out of business). I was now in search of a new position and was very pre-occupied with that process, as well as my painful hip. I discovered I could still ride the bicycle on the paved bike path from Lake Dillon to the top of Vail Pass and back, about a forty mile ride with, roughly, a three thousand foot change in elevation. Driving a car, however, was becoming too painful, even with the collection of cushions I was starting to pile up to sit on.

Having a pre-scheduled vacation trip to Hawaii, I and my wife, Mary Lou, proceeded with our plans. Two things really stood out, in my mind, during this trip:

First, it was the first time visiting Hawaii that I did not pick up a surfboard. I knew I would not be able to swing my right leg up onto the board to paddle out, let alone get up onto the board after catching a wave. This was certainly a sign that my hip was really bothering me. I was increasingly becoming less able to "muscle" my way through this.

The second striking memory of that trip was the tremendous pain that would awake me every morning about two am. On most occasions, I would "hobble" outside to the hot tub for a soak. On one occasion, I was on my back, floating on the bubbles, looking at the stars. I was totally supported by the hot tub bubbles and slightly bending my body, in different positions, to ease pressure on the nerves that were possibly being pinched, as in "classic sciatica." Unable to find any type of floating position that relieved the pain, I suddenly had the thought that "*this might be cancer.*" I still have no idea why "cancer" came into my mind, as I knew so little about it.

I tried to suppress that thought, and did not even mention it to my orthopedic physician when I saw him for my July 19th appointment. He, too, thought this was still my sciatica, although it had progressed longer than usual. He suggested a shot of cortisone directly near a nerve that he suspected was the problem. I lay down on the table, he loaded a syringe, and gave me a mighty "big and bad feeling" injection.

My son, Greg, happened to be in town, passing through from Chicago, on his way to Las Vegas to attend school. I found him asleep in his car, in my driveway, about four that morning. He drove me to the orthopedic clinic and was waiting for me outside in the car, not surprisingly, asleep again. I hobbled out and he woke up, looked at me, and his eyes grew bright as he sensed my pain and asked if I was alright. I told him—*"I think I just got a brick put into my hip."* It was mighty sore!

My orthopedic physician said if I did not have relief in two days to come back to try a shot in another area. I was back in two days without relief. This time I watched as he started loading the syringe, which now looked as though it was the size for veterinary use, and explained the "brick in my hip" feeling two days before.

I said: *"I don't feel good about this."*

He replied: *"Oh yea, these things hurt like hell—don't they?"*

I said, with conviction: *"yes they do! But what I mean—is that something is wrong—all the physical therapy, all the medications, time, and the shot have not produced one bit of relief. Something just feels really wrong."*

My orthopedic physician, knowing he had treated me for my injured neck for a number of years, asked if we ever looked at my lower back. I assured him we had not, as I have never had a lower back problem. He decided to have an X-ray taken by his radiology technician. Twenty minutes later, I was back in they exam room. The orthopedic physician came in, and, as he put the first X-ray onto the light box, he immediately turned to me, somewhat startled, and asked:

"Why is your L-4 vertebrae so white?"

Thinking he was joking, I replied with a chuckle:

"I thought maybe you would know."

His demeanor turned very serious:

He said: *"No! I don't!"*

"But we need to find out what this is. We need to rule out a pagetoid process or something."

He decided to bring in one of his partners to take a look, and he also said it was suggestive of Paget's disease, although unusual for only one vertebrae to have it. My orthopedic physician, sitting in front of me, said:

"lets get a myelogram and CT done."

He patted me on the leg and said: *"don't worry, we will find out what's giving you all this pain."*

I went in for a myelogram and CT scan at the medical imaging center, August 9th, where I had the facet blocks done, back in May. I was starting to realize for a patient, it seems a lot of time passes by when waiting for medical appointments. The first technician I spoke with was preparing me for the myelogram and making small talk about my dark sun tan. When I told him I just returned from vacation on the big Island of Hawaii, he explained that he used to go to the big island as punishment when he misbehaved. He lived on the island of Maui, but his father was stationed on the army base along saddleback road.

His only memory of the big island, therefore, was an army base out in the black lava desert with no ocean in site! No wonder he did not care for the Big Island!

The interventional radiologist came in and made some small talk—the kind of small talk, I believe, is made with most patients he sees. As he put my spine X-rays from the orthopedic clinic up onto the light box he said:

"Off hand, this does not look like Paget's. It looks more like a tumor, but the kind that is rarely ever cancerous."

We proceeded with the myelogram. This procedure involves inserting a needle into the small of the back, into an opening between two vertebrae, and into to the spinal canal. A dye is inserted into the spinal canal, and a fluoroscope screen made it all visible to me. He first showed me the catheter insertion on the screen. In a calm voice, he continued to explain exactly what he was doing. He showed me that I had plenty of room in the spinal canal, and commented, *"this is a good thing."* He stopped talking to me and instructed the technician to start tilting the table and start taking "pictures" of the spinal area. Tilting the table takes advantage of gravity and forces the dye to travel up or down the spine, according to the tilt of the table. I asked how it looked, and in somewhat of a stern voice, the radiologist said:

"I can't tell much from the screen, there is more detail from the actual film shots we are taking."

In a more concerned voice, he asked who my orthopedic surgeon was, and when I told him, he said:

"Good, he is good, and is conservative when it comes to actual surgery."

I think this was my first clue that something might be really wrong with my spine. When the procedure was finished, the radiologist put his hand on my shoulder, and in a very sincere tone said:

"Don't worry. We are putting together a very good set of pictures for your orthopedic surgeon"

This was my second clue that something was wrong!

I was wheeled into the CT scan room, in a wheel chair, due to the invasive nature of the myelogram. It was cold in the room, and I started to shiver and shake, all the while thinking of those two odd clues from the radiologist who performed the myelogram procedure. The CT technician came in and immediately gave me a blanket. She asked why I was there, and we made the usual small talk, again, I imagined the kind she has with most patients she sees, as I got up onto the table. She was friendly and in a seemingly happy mood. When I was in place for the scan, she went out into the control room, and soon the whirring sound of the machine started. In a short time, it stopped and the technician came back into the room.

In a somewhat startled tone she asked:

"Have you had major lower back surgery in the past?"

I replied, *"No, why does it look like it?"*

She quite calmly, as if correcting herself, said:

"Ah-no, I was just wondering."

She went back to the control room and we finished the scan. When the scan was finished, she too had changed her demeanor from very pleasant and happy, to one of concern and seriousness. With another empathetic pat on my shoulder, I left the CT scan room. To me this was my third clue that, not only was something not right, but was really wrong! The thought of something life threatening, however, had not yet entered my mind.

Time Line: 2001: February, March, April, May, June, July, August

On August 10, my orthopedic physician called, telling me that the radiologist from the medical imaging center had called and described what he saw was a "smoldering" L-4 vertebrae. This, as my orthopedic physician explained, meant there was something wrong, and the vertebrae was just the *"smoke from an already fired gun."* He already had ordered a bone scan and said *"I want to see every bone in your body."* He also wanted a biopsy of the L-4 vertebrae, and anything else that might show up on the scan. He added that he had not yet seen the reports or the pictures, but said:

"I am concerned and I do not mind letting you know."

On August 15, I pre-registered at the local hospital. I took comfort going to this particular hospital, as it was literally 4-5 blocks from our house, and it is where I had my pacemaker inserted. When I pre-registered, I was told I needed to bring in my X-rays, myelogram, CT scan films, and corresponding reports. I contacted the medical imaging center to pick these up. I picked them up, drove home and laid them on the dinning room table while I looked for my reading glasses. The big envelopes were sealed shut, but I wanted to take a look at the films and read the reports that, I was told, were inside. I put my glasses on, and immediately noticed that someone had written on the outside of the X-ray envelope, and underlined the word:

"Malignant"

This was the first time someone had "spelled out" or even mentioned that word to me, and it was a "punch in the stomach." I knew something was wrong, but the word "malignant" really wasn't in my vocabulary of self descriptors!

In the corresponding report, inside the film envelope, the radiologist wrote he was "very uncomfortable with a malignant looking mass in the L-4 vertebrae." I was feeling a little panicky, but quickly realized this is what we had been looking for. That is really what I thought floating on the bubbles in the hot tub in Hawaii five months before. Seeing the word "malignant" made it real,—very real—very quickly. However, I was now beginning to see something I could focus on, and deal with.

In order to see if I had any similar "spots" in other bones, I had a full body bone scan on August 20. This consisted of receiving an injection of material that was "tagged" radioactively, wait for a couple of hours, then lay on a table for about 45 minutes while a machine slowly scanned my entire skeletal structure. It was an easy test, and I was assured that my results would be available for the next day's biopsy. As simple as the test is, it is very sensitive to any metabolic abnormality. For example, a "hair line" crack that would not show up on an X-ray, would show up on this type of bone scan.

On August 21, I checked into outpatient surgery for the biopsy. I began to feel stress because time was going by slowly, in terms of medical appointments. This was in contrast to what I have seen in the movies. In "movie land", when someone is suspected of having cancer, they are admitted to the hospital, surgery is performed, a biopsy is done, and they are on chemotherapy and/or radiation within a couple of days. I started this medical journey in April. Already five months had gone by and we were still trying to diagnose what my "problem" was.

Based on the previous day's bone scan, I was first taken to X-ray. The technicians said the interventional radiologist first wanted to X-ray my right femur (upper leg) and my left humerus (upper arm). One technician said I may not need a biopsy, based on the X-rays. The interventional radiologist spoke with me after he had seen the X-rays, said that it looked like the femur and humerus had Paget's disease, and that the medical imaging center's films of the L-4 vertebrae did not look like Paget's. Instead, it looked like a non-cancerous tumor in the bone. He had another radiologist take a look at the X-rays, and they both decided that I had Paget's disease in my leg and arm, and a non-cancerous tumor in the L-4 vertebrae. Their advice was to skip the biopsy and begin treatment for Paget's.

After thinking about it for a couple of minutes, I stated that it would be difficult to go home and "move forward" without getting the biopsy, after getting a suspected malignancy report on the L-4 vertebrae. They agreed and decided to perform the biopsy, and it was "onward" to the procedure.

The physician performing the biopsy explained that it would be impossible to get to the "sweet spot" in my L-4 vertebrae, as I had a "vascular lake" in the center of it. The "sweet spot" was the center of controversy. This is where the X-ray and CT films showed "something"—either non-cancerous, or cancerous activity. He said he would get as close to "hitting" this "spot" as he could. He explained, however, the "sweet spot" was in the front portion of the L-4 vertebrae, and with all the space and organs he would have to get through with a bone core instrument, it would be impossible to get at.

Even though I was sedated well for the procedure, I remember the force the radiologist used to pull out the plug of bone from my L-4 vertebrae. It was as though, while lying on my stomach, someone picked me off the table by pulling my belt. He let out a grunt of exertion and my mid section came back to the table were I was face to face with a masked nurse.

I asked her: *"was that the biopsy?"*

She said: *"yes it was!"*

I noticed two people bent over and working at a lab bench. They checked out the bone sample and said it was good to run all of the tests on. Results would be ready within forty-eight hours.

It was August 24, and I expected results the day before, but they were not available. My orthopedic physician called me to ask if I had the biopsy performed. I confirmed, and he told me he was anxious to get a report. He went on to say he had spoken with my primary care physician and the radiologist from the medical imaging center. I told him that I was concerned, as I had read the radiology report regarding a "possible malignancy."

After a pause, my orthopedic physician said: *"I've got to tell you, my heart stopped when I saw that."*

He said he would call me as soon as he got the report from the biopsy. I went into another weekend without a lot of information, other than I had a sore hip.

My daughter Kelly had been calling quite frequently. She was frightened about me having a biopsy. She calls often and comes right out and says how frightened she is, and feels isolated because she now lives and works on the East Coast. Greg does not express his concern, but I speak with him more often, as he was going to school and living in Las Vegas. I told both Kelly and Greg, that the results of the biopsy did not matter, as whatever it is, I will just get the appropriate treatment. As always, I believe they have taken on my positive attitude.

On August 27, my orthopedic called and said the findings all pointed to Paget's disease. He said he was relieved, and knew I was too.

3

Paget's Disease

Time Line: 2001: February, March, April, May, June, July, August, September

Principle 4: Be An Involved Life Long Learner

In September, I started researching Paget's disease on the Internet. Paget's disease of the bone is a chronic skeletal disorder that often results in enlarged or deformed bones in one or more regions of the skeleton. Excessive bone breakdown and formation of new bone can result in bone that is dense but fragile. Pain is the most common symptom. Complications may include arthritis, fractures, bowing of limbs, and hearing loss if Paget's disease affects the skull. Though the causes are not known, medical therapies are available to manage the disease. The disease is more prevalent in the UK, Australia, and the New England states of the U.S. I have some English ancestry, on my mother's side, but I did not think enough to have what I felt was an "English" disease. All I knew was that I had pain in my hip that I really wanted to go away, and I was relived that I did not have cancer.

I also looked for U.S. experts in treating Paget's disease. I was surprised to learn that the two most often Internet cited physicians treating Paget's, were in Denver, Colorado. I was feeling very positive to learn this information, and called their office to learn more of their practice.

On September 15, I was back to see my orthopedic surgeon. Again, he expressed his relief that this was not "something more serious." He started talking of Paget's disease, that no one dies of Paget's, and that he wasn't sure how to treat it. In fact, he admitted, this was the first case of Paget's he had ever seen, and that none of the other nine orthopedics in the clinic had ever seen a case. I offered my research and the physicians' names that were "Paget's experts," and that they were in Denver. He was aware of one name and said *"she is an up and coming bone specialist I've heard of"* and called her office to set up an appointment for me.

Principle 5: Find A Coach

My first encounter with the endocrinologist bone specialist, on October 1, was very positive. Dr. Carol is a runner and, as I sensed quickly, has an "unstoppable attitude." Right away, I was impressed with how she communicated with me. I knew there would be no lack of real information from her. She completed a very thorough exam of me. I realized, even with all of the talk of cancer the past few months, that was the first thorough check for swollen lymph nodes.

I had a bone density test performed in her office, and she said she suspected that I also had osteoporosis. She sent me to a local lab for blood tests, and scheduled an immediate dose of Aredia®, a treatment for both Paget's and osteoporosis (at a lower dosage). Aredia® is an IV drug, and it was going to be administered back at the hospital, in the cancer department. Later, researching Aredia, I found that it was used quite often in breast cancer, when the cancer had metastasized into the bone. There, again, was another "strange" connection with cancer.

On October 11, I received my first IV dose of Aredia®, which lasted about five and one half hours. It was my first visit to any kind of cancer treatment center. What I remember so vividly was how out of place I was. I was witness to people with cancer, receiving chemotherapy drugs to save their lives. There were people sick, people without hair, and accompanying family members that looked more concerned than the patients. Then there was me. I felt like an imposter! I had some kind of bone disease, and I was a very active Ironman®, and, most importantly, I did not have cancer. I felt like such an intruder into those peoples' suffering. That night, I thought about the sickness that cancer patients often suffer, as I endured some very minor flu like symptoms from the Aredia®.

October 19 marked my second dose of Aredia®. It lasted about five hours. I was having more pain in my hip, and now my lower back. I again was thinking how medicine moved so slow in reality, as opposed to the swiftness shown in the movies. I found out, however from Dr. Carol, that she suspected "something" other than Paget's disease. Being proactive with my case, she had sent out copies of my records, X-rays, CT scans, and myelograms to experts in New York, St. Louis, and the Mayo Clinic in Minnesota. She also put me on crutches for three months. As she explained, the Aredia® would turn my femur to a very fragile state, and the last thing she wanted was for me to break my leg, as a broken femur, whether Paget's, cancer, or osteoporosis, would be a very serious thing. I took her coaching advice seriously, and stayed off the leg.

I was still concerned with the time rolling along. I mentioned to Dr. Carol that the medical world seemed to work in reverse of "dog" years. What one would think should take one week, seems to take seven weeks. She, has since, explained to me that the patient and the physician experience time in different ways. She and other physicians are often very aware and sometimes embarrassed by the agonizing long duration of time between the presentation of a person's symptoms and the actual final diagnosis. When a diagnosis is particularly difficult, as was mine, multiple opinions are sought from physicians who are not personally involved and do not share the same time pressure to provide opinions. Rightfully so, I am sure they are primarily focused on their own patients. Physicians, like their patients are also frustrated and anxious about the process!

On October 24, Dr. Carol called to provide an update on the specialists she had sent my records to. Wow! More than a great physician, she is a great coach! She actually called me to share information, giving me feedback and advice on next actions to take! For the most part, the response, from the experts was "looks like an interesting case." She wanted to remind me to stay on crutches for the three months. She was not worried about the current pain, as she was about the possibility of feeling well enough to "test" my fragile right leg. I was scheduled for another blood test for her evaluation. I was feeling that, with this coach, I was making progress on the treatments. I was also feeling that I was starting to make progress on landing a job. Basically, I was making progress on the two outstanding "difficult" issues in my life.

By November, I had also been having a pain in my left leg that seemed like a type of neuropathy. To me, it was definitely some nerve involvement, not bone. Dr Carol wanted me to see a neurologist, to get an EMG—not one of my favorite tests in the world.

The neurologist first checked me out by lifting my left leg, and created an amazingly sharp pain, to which I reacted with a quick recoil and a verbal *"ouch."* I remembered that my orthopedic had also done the same thing, and I wish I had thought of telling the neurologist, before hand.

On November 5th, Dr Carol called to tell me that The University of Colorado Health Science Center had re-stained the hospital biopsy slides and came to the conclusion there was no Paget's disease, and the biopsy was also negative for cancer. She had not heard from the expert in St. Louis, but she had spoken with a number of other physicians. She went on to tell me that it almost looked as though my bones had outgrown their vascular capability—something that is seen with severe trauma to the bone. She had also spoken with my orthopedic physician about setting up another biopsy and CT scan to check the progression, if any. I reminded her that the interventional radiologist that performed the original biopsy said he could not get to the place in my L-4 vertebrae that he "really wanted to get to" because of a "vascular lake" in the vertebrae.

She had not forgotten about the difficulty getting to the "sweet" spot in my vertebrae. She was my coach, and knew my case. She said for that very reason she wanted to see another biopsy. She also asked about my pain, and I told her it was getting progressively worse:

"I'm only getting three hours a sleep at a time, before I need to get up for pain pills"

She told me to stay on the crutches, and that the Aredia® should have made me feel better by this time. It works that way, *"Not always, but usually."* She said my orthopedic physician would schedule everything at my neighborhood hospital and that I would hear from him.

I had put in a couple of telephone calls to my orthopedic physicians' scheduling department, after the discussion with Dr Carol, to get the CT scan and biopsy scheduled. They had heard nothing from my orthopedic physician, as he had been out of town for a couple of days. My orthopedic physician called around eleven the morning of November 7th, and said he had spoken with Dr Carol about getting the CT scan and biopsy scheduled. I reminded him about the interventional radiologist's difficulties in getting at the "sweet" spot.

He replied that the pathologist and he had already spoken about getting the biopsy from the femur, but they did not want to weaken it, and that the vertebrae actually provided an easier access to the bone. He also said they also agreed that it was probably the same process going on in my femur as the L-4 vertebrae.

On November 9th, the orthopedic scheduler was having difficulty getting approval from my insurance company. I stated the reason for that was I have a new insurance company. Under my new insurance, I needed a referral from my primary care physician. I immediately called my primary care physician's referral person, and explained that I needed a referral for a CT scan and biopsy. She asked what the reason was and I replied *"I assume we are trying to rule out cancer."* The CT scan was finally approved and scheduled for November 26, 2001, and the biopsy was scheduled for December 6th, 2001.

As I lay on the CT scan table on November 26th, I again was finding the length of time it took to get this test and the biopsy test scheduled for December 6, pretty incredibly long. Again I had only my experience watching television and movies that normally make diagnosing cancer a pretty urgent and fast thing to do. I also had my left humerus X-rayed for Dr Carol. While I was at the hospital,

I spoke with the radiology nurse about pre-registering for the December 6th biopsy. I mentioned the difficulty in diagnosing the "spot" in my vertebrae, and she said that Paget's looked many different ways, but that is probably what it was.

I spoke with Dr Carol on December 3rd, and asked about the CT scan results. She said it showed no change and *"that is not good."* She reminded me to make sure the upcoming biopsy report should be sent to her, in addition to my orthopedic physician, and she wanted the University of Colorado Health Science Center pathologists to read the slides, in addition to my hospital pathologists. I mentioned to her the time lag in trying to get these things done. With true empathy, she agreed, but thought I was doing a good job expediting things. I flat out asked her what we are looking for, and she told me that they wanted to clarify the diagnosis and look again for a tumor. She said, *"it still could be Paget's, but we want to make sure."*

My orthopedic physician also called, later in the evening, and I asked:

"What exactly are we looking for in the biopsy—cancer?"

He compassionately stumbled with his words and said:

"Well, no, ah, well, the diagnosis needs to be clarified." He went on to say that *"Dr Carol and her endochrinology "cronies" needed to verify the Paget's diagnosis."* I was continuously becoming a bigger and bigger fan of Dr Carol, my endocrinologist "coach."

Before the biopsy, on December 6th, I was again wheeled into the X-ray room for pictures of my femurs, my left arm, and my vertebrae. I was then prepped for the biopsy. During my previous biopsy, I had found this to be a somewhat brutal procedure, both mentally and physically. The fact that I had been through this procedure recently, did not help. The same nurses involved with today's biopsy remembered me from the first. The same doctor explained the procedure, and I said: *"yes, I remember, especially when you pulled the bone core sample out of my back."*

He said: *"Oh, you can't remember that, you were too far sedated."*

So I turned to the nurse, and I asked: *"do you remember when I asked if that was the biopsy—when the Doctor pulled me up off the table and I fell back on it?"*

She exclaimed, to everyone in the room: *"Wow, he does remember!"*

After that, I was "really" sedated—I do not remember one thing of this biopsy procedure!

I made a startling discovery on December 10th. I realized with my short sleep periods, and my getting up throughout the night to take another pain pill, that I had been taking six to eight times the recommended dose. I immediately decided to back down to one tablet every eight to twelve hours. I also realized the

Aredia® medication treatments were working, as now I really hurt in my right leg, my right hip, and now even into my shin.

I was no longer worried about the diagnosis, as I was becoming more concerned that there may not be one. I can easily face known challenges. It is the unknowns that are much more difficult!

I called the local hospital on December 13th, and spoke with a radiology nurse who immediately recognized my name.

I said: *"I have two questions for you, first, when will the biopsy reports be released to my orthopedic and my endochrinologist physicians?"*

She told me that only the gross report was done and the final report would be sent out that afternoon. I realized my second question was to again state that a copy needed to be sent to my endochrinologist physician, and the nurse replied, *"Oh, yes, she called yesterday to find out where the report is."* Again, Dr. Carol is the one, of my many doctors, who stayed on top of things and gave me confidence that some answers will be arriving in my immediate future.

I put in calls into both my orthopedic and Dr. Carol on December 14th. I just wanted to hear any kind of a diagnosis. By now I did not think it was cancer, but I really needed some kind of label for what ever was going on. Only then could I accept it and treat it. I knew I would be up to the challenge of dealing with, and winning over whatever the diagnosis would be—just give me one. It was Friday, and I headed into the weekend without hearing from my physicians.

On December 17th, Dr. Carol left a telephone voice mail. She said the hospital that did the biopsy had not received the results back from the "sample that was sent to the Mayo Clinic." She said it as though I knew it had been sent to Mayo. It was, however, the first I heard about it. She also said the X-rays showed no increase and that was a good thing. I still had no diagnosis, and I increasingly wanted one.

On December 19th, Dr. Carol called from her home and said she had just received the report from Mayo Clinic. A pathologist at Mayo was one of the world's experts in bone pathology. The results, as Dr. Carol went on to say, showed that they could not rule out Paget's, but also cannot rule out cancer. The Mayo pathologist had found a couple of cells that looked cancerous, but needed more material to make a final determination. Dr. Carol asked about my pain, and told me that if it was cancer, the first step in treatment would be the same Aredia® that I was already receiving. So even if I was feeling that I was losing time, she assured me that I had not been losing real significant time.

I was now convinced there were two different medical times. One is "patient time," the other is "physician time." It is the waiting that was driving me crazy. It had now been about nine months since I had seen a physician about my "sore hip." I was becoming aware this was a "tough case," but I still wanted a diagnosis to focus on—and I wanted it soon! As I previously stated, Dr. Carol was also acutely aware of the time passing.

I put a call into my orthopedic physician regarding biopsy questions. I really wanted to know the next steps. Instead, I received a call that evening from the head pathologist from the hospital where I had my biopsy done. He said he just wanted to let me know what was going on, as he was aware I had been waiting for a report "too long." He said he just sent all of my X-rays and CT Scans to the pathologist at the Mayo Clinic in Minnesota. The problem in getting a new biopsy sample, as Mayo requested, would be very severe surgery, going directly through the abdomen. He had spoken with my orthopedic surgeon, who said that this kind of surgery might have too high a risk factor to try it for "just" a biopsy.

So, the current solution, as the radiologist told me, was to send all of my films to the bone pathologist at Mayo.

"*He is the worlds best bone pathologist,*" the hospital radiologist said, "*and he is going to look at your films, in addition to your biopsy we sent to him, and make a determination if it is cancer or not.*" "*If he cannot figure it out, you should wait and see what happens.*"

I replied how long I already had been waiting to see what happens. He replied:

"*If this is a cancer, I would guess it will be a bone lymphoma, and I am aware of at least one pro-athlete that had it and recovered from it. This would be very treatable.*"

He said to give him a call on Friday, towards the end of the day, and provided his cell number. He added he would be out of the country for the weekend, and if one of his associates received the report from the Mayo pathologist, they had instructions to pass on the information immediately to Dr. Carol and my orthopedic physician.

My orthopedic physician called on December 20, and asked me to bring in the very first set of CT scan films from the medical imaging center. He said:

"*In view of the information that there is not any change, I think we should sit on this instead of trying such a drastic procedure as an open biopsy from the front.*" He went on to explain he had spoken with a number of his partners, and "*none of them recommends such a drastic surgery on an otherwise healthy individual.*"

I also commented that my pain was a bit worse, and he admitted that he always forgets that part. He also said he was taking my records to a local medical conference on spinal surgery the next week.

On December 21st, I dropped all of the X-ray and CT films I had been collecting, for sometime, to my orthopedics' office. I also gave the local hospital pathologist a call, and he said he had not heard from Mayo. I sensed during this conversation that he already had one foot out of the country. Meanwhile, it was pain as usual, and with the holiday coming up, I was giving up reason to think I would know more before the end of the year.

On December 24th, I called the local hospital pathologist only to find out that he had not heard from the Mayo pathologist.

Principle 6: Be A Coach

On December 26, I received good news in the form of a job offer. It sounded like an interesting one, too. It was with the Small Business Administration, as a Director of a particular piece of geography in the northern suburbs of Denver. Better yet, my office would be hosted by Westminster Community College. I enjoy the campus atmosphere, and I was looking forward to being part of it, and get some healing done at the same time. I also knew it would be a good environment in which to heal the femur of my right leg. I would also be able to continue my adjunct teaching at the University of Colorado, Denver Campus, where I had been teaching marketing classes in the Undergraduate and Graduate Schools of Business. The University of Colorado was my official "coaching" position and I was pleased and proud to teach at least one class a semester for the last four years at the University campus.

Now, I more than ever, wanted to know something so I can aggressively "deal" with it, and start my new position and get things moving. I was sure I would hear about the results from Mayo, and also from my orthopedic surgeon regarding the spinal surgery conference he was attending the next day.

The orthopedic physician called to say he had discussed my case with other local orthopedic doctors and they agreed with him and his partners. Basically, no one wanted to perform an open biopsy through my front side, particularly on such an "otherwise healthy" person. He went on to say that he also spoke with two "tumor doctors." My orthopedic physician, during the entire adventure never used the terms "oncologist", or "cancer". Being a very "compassionate" physician, I think he just had a difficult time using those words with his patients.

He said he had received the Mayo Clinic report and it was "non-specific." It stated it may represent some lymphoma, but it *could not be determined.* The local oncologists told him even if he were able to get into the "sweet" spot, inside the L-4 vertebrae, *you won't find anything.* They did, however suggest another blood metabolism workup, including a PSA, and CT Scans of the chest, abdomen, and pelvis. I believed Dr Carol, my endochrinologist, had previously run the PSA and the blood metabolism workup. I did not mention this, as I thought it might be an interesting comparison. The CT Scan was scheduled for the next day, December 27th. I thought, *"The next day?" "Wow, now we are moving ahead!"*

The purpose of this CT scan was to look for any lymphomas in any place, other than my bones. The idea was that Lymphoma normally strikes soft tissue first, particularly lymph nodes (hence the name lymphoma cancer). When it is not treated or is untreatable, the cancer will often metastasize and spread to another area—usually soft tissue, and lastly into the bone. So the rationale was if we could identify a cancer in the soft tissue, we would know for sure if it was cancer in the L-4 vertebrae.

This was my first CT Scan that I drank contrast media for, as well as received an IV hook up for an iodine based imaging media. The iodine created an immediate taste in my mouth, as it is quickly metabolized in the lungs. I was amazed how fast it occurs. From the IV entry into my lower arm, to the time I could taste it was less than the time for the technician to tell me: *"you will have a funny metallic taste in your mouth very quickly."*

As soon as he got to the word *"funny"*—I tasted it. After the usual scan, the technician came into the room to say they wanted a "delayed shot."

The technician, upon completing the scan, asked if I had a CT before, and I replied that Mary Lou and I had just been talking about the feeling of being in the movie "Ground Hog Day." *"Yes," I said. "I have been in this machine, without the contrast dye and media, about four times in the last few months."* He said physicians could call for the gross results on Friday, but the final written report would be sent to them on Monday.

I found out from my twin sister, Sue, that my father's brother, Freddie, had died at the age of twenty-seven, from Hodgkin's Lymphoma. So much for having no family history of cancer!

It was now Monday, December 31st—the day of "complete knowledge." I called the local hospital to see about the CT scan, and they had "no report on file." The technician on the telephone said, *"Since it isn't filed, it hasn't been done."* I was truly amazed. Wouldn't they rush writing a report that was crucial to a diagnosis of cancer? My stress level, closing out the year without knowing anything, was very difficult.

_Time Line__: 2001: February, March, April, May, June, July, August, September, October, November, December_
_Time Line__: 2002: January_

I started the New Year off the way 2001 ended, it seemed. I called Dr. Carol's office and left a voicemail stating that I still had no results from the hospital for the CT scan. I was feeling a lot of stress, as I had not been exercising, except for an arm workout using the crutches. I had a new job to start pretty soon, and wanted to put all of the illness behind me. Dr. Carol called on the evening of January 2nd. She too, was baffled by the hospital still not having the CT scan report finished and available. She really caught my attention, however when she said I could start carefully going off the crutches! She also asked for some X-rays that the orthopedic physician had, and I said I would pick them up and deliver them to her office. She wanted to send them to a radiologist in St. Louis, the "world's bone X-ray expert."

On January 3rd, the records department at the local hospital confirmed the report was finished and they would send it to my orthopedic and Dr Carol "right away."

I called my orthopedic physician's office on January 4th, to find out about the test results. I was surprised, but more disappointed to find out the hospital had not sent out the report. I put in three more calls to the records department, each time leaving a voice mail. In the late afternoon, I finally connected with a "live" person who said she would find out about my CT scan report and call me back. She never did, and I felt extremely slighted, crushed, and left out dangling at the mercy of someone who did not care that my CT scan report was now three days late.

I started another 24 hour urine test Dr Carol wanted me to complete. I also put in a call to the local hospital on January 7th and spoke with the same records person I had spoken to before. She said _"oh, we found the notes and they will be dictated and sent to your physicians today."_ I am not sure what she meant by "found" my notes. I just wanted to move things along. So far, it seemed that my biggest wait times have been scheduling and obtaining reports from my local hospital.

My orthopedic called and said the CT scan report showed the chest and abdomen were clear, and while there were no enlarged lymph nodes, I seemed to have an abnormally large quantity of lymph nodes in the pelvic region. He had already spoken with my primary care physician to refer me to an oncologist. He said _"let's clear this red herring up once and for all."_

Dr. Carol, my endocrinologist, also called and gave the oncologist I would be seeing "high marks." She said she knew of him, having done her residency the same year and same place he completed his. I dropped off all the X-rays and various scans at her office. She wanted to speak to me, so I waited a short while. All she had to say was what she had been suspecting all along, and championed my case to my other physicians to "keep at it." She said:

"Its looking more and more like this isn't Paget's."

On January 10th, the local hospital pathologist called and apologized that no one from the hospital had called me about the Mayo clinic report over the holidays. I "filled" him in on the appointment made for me with the oncologist, and his response was:

"He is the right guy to see—he is one of the best!" The pathologist said he would call the oncologist to provide his input on the case.

January 15th marked my long awaited appointment with the highly recommended oncologist. I first went into a room with two nurses, and they explained how chemo therapy was given, some of the side effects, etc. I was really feeling low, as they caught me by surprise. I was not even thinking of chemotherapy. After all, no one had yet said I had cancer.

I went into one of the patient "holding" rooms and waited for the oncologist. He came in, carrying my stack of films and reports and looked very surprised. In a very forceful voice, he said:

"I can tell you right now that you do not have cancer!" *"Well, It's always possible you might have a minor lymphoma, but if you had cancer, with these CT Scans and X-rays, you should at the very least look like a prisoner of war."*

He went on to explain that every few years a patient like me comes along with "ugly" looking CT scans and X-rays. Their films, records, and biopsy slides are sent around the country to all the experts, and everyone forgets to "look at the patient." He said:

"It's obvious you do not have cancer. You are just plain too healthy looking."

He, somewhat angrily, explained more reasoning:

"If you had cancer," he went on, *"There could be two types."* *"The first, and you would have already been dead."* *"That's what your films look like, but obviously you are here!"* (Actually I knew he was speaking of osteo sarcoma, and I was aware that I had already lived too long with an undiagnosed case of this type of cancer. One of the physicians, during a CT scan about 6 months into the diagnosis project remarked, with a chuckle, *"Well, I guess it isn't what it looks like!"*).

"The second," the oncologist went on: *"and I doubt you have it, is very treatable lymphoma—even six months from now."*

He said the open biopsy surgery had "ten times" the risk of having this second cancer for six months, and to re-take the CT Scans at that time.

"In the meantime," he said *"I think you have Paget's disease and you should continue on treatment for that."*

I walked out of that oncology clinic feeling like an intruder. The oncologist, I felt, almost threw me out of his clinic because I did not have cancer. I was feeling good, on the other hand, to be thrown out because I did not have cancer and, again, I felt I had Paget's disease. I was most anxious to start my new job, and get on with treatment for Paget's disease.

I had a January 29th appointment with Dr. Carol who informed me the bone "markers" were down, indicating the Aredia® had finally shown a result. However, the twenty-four hour urine test showed I was leaking calcium more than the previous test. She had spoken with the oncologist about setting up another CT scan in six months. She was still persistent in getting some answers about my case, and I was appreciating her efforts. I, however, was feeling that cancer was out of the picture. Dr. Carol's partner met with an expert in St. Louis to discuss my case. His assessment was a familiar one received from the experts: "this is an interesting case."

Dr. Carol was now the sole adventurer in my case, and she had much empathy regarding my long effort to find out what was going on. My hip and leg were actually feeling quite a bit better by now. She now had a very thick file of correspondence from other physicians, lab tests, and CT scan reports. She started me on Moduretic®, a combination of amiloride and hydrochlorothiazide. Amiloride is a potassium sparing diuretic that also inhibits calcium excretion. Her idea was to "force" the calcium back to the bones, where it was "supposed to be."

I expressed to her, my concern about my L-4 vertebrae, since it was looking to be in bad shape in all of the CT Scans. She assured me I had enough muscle mass to support it. Her concern, however, was still my right femur.

She said: *"it still has a high risk of breaking."* "In addition," she continued, *"I am concerned about the soft tissue around the vertebrae that looks bad."* This was my first knowledge of that, and I wondered why no one else had mentioned it before. After all, my endochrinologist is not an orthopedic surgeon, nor an oncologist, yet she was always leading the charge, particularly with information. I confess, I was getting tired of the process of finding out, and was willing to accept the Paget's diagnosis, just to "move on." She was not. While I was feeling "dropped" through the institutional "cracks" of medical testing, appointments, scheduling, reporting, etc., she stayed on my "case."

She also had a discussion with the oncologist that I saw. From what she told me, it sounded as though he still thought there could be a cancer, but that an operation that was required to obtain a biopsy was too risky. The best thing, he said, was to recheck with new CT scans in six months. I stopped by my primary care physician's office for the "monthly blood workup."

In March I was beginning to feel much better. I had started at my new job, was off crutches, and took advantage of a one quarter mile long hallway at the college to take a couple of walks each day. There was also a swimming pool that was a short walk from my office to swim laps during lunch or early morning. My previous thought was correct, "this was a good environment to heal." While my body was feeling better, and I was having much less pain, I was extremely fatigued. I taught early morning business classes on the campus, but drove to two other campuses every other week for a noontime class, and a night class. In addition, I taught my twice-weekly night graduate class at the University of Colorado. So I attributed the fatigue to my hours, and my re-introduction to some exercise.

After a couple of calls to my primary care physician's office on March 13th, I managed to get my blood report from the test done, January 26th. I was somewhat amazed by the length of time to obtain the report. The results showed everything was "normal," which was consistently normal throughout my medical history. In addition, I was pretty convinced that I had no cancer, and the Aredia® had worked on the Paget's disease. I felt my life was starting to get back to "normal."

"Normalcy" was short lived. By March 19th, I started to note some symptoms, although I still associated them with the long hours I was gladly putting in, (mostly to feel I was "making up" for my unemployment time) and my increase in exercise, mostly swimming. I was waking in the early morning hours, one or two o'clock, with low back and tail bone pain. Every once in a while I was also feeling pain in my right femur. I thought that I was possible having a flare up of the Paget's, and maybe I was due for an infusion of Aredia®. I was also experiencing a periodic night sweating episode, as well as some strange itching.

One year had passed, since I started to seek medical help. On April 1st, I provided blood for my monthly "normal" check, and also a twenty four hour urine sample. I was doing more research on the Internet and became strongly suspicious that I had a problem or benign tumor in one of my parathyroid glands that would have been a cause of drawing calcium out of the bones. When I suggested this to Dr. Carol, I knew I had become "one of those" patients that come up with weird or obscure diseases for themselves. She kindly explained why I did not have this particular disease, and I embarrassingly listened to the scientific rationale. I relied on her to be my coach and "captain" my case, and realized she had considered and thought through this and many other explanations of my symptoms.

I was having quite a bit of "heart burn" or GERD (gastric esophageal reflux disorder). I was taking 6 X 250mg of Naprosyn® every day. Upon waking up one night with acid in my throat, I decided "that" was enough of "that!" But overall, things were O.K. Cancer was basically "gone" from my mind, and I was treating Paget's disease every two-three months with an infusion of Aredia®.

I re-visited the medical imaging center on July 9th, to have another look at my L-4 vertebrae, and the lymph nodes in my body. The interventional radiologist was the same physician that performed the facet blocks on my neck back in May, 2001. He performed the myelogram and showed me on the screen, as he narrated:

"As you can see," "Things are pretty tight in there"

I could easily make out the definite constriction of my spinal cord, within the L-4 vertebrae. I knew from his thirty second hand shake and his sincere wishes of *"best of everything to you,"* that "things" truly had gotten worse. I already knew the pain was returning to my hip, lower back and right femur. The results of the myelogram showed a soft tissue mass was compressing the spinal cord and it made sense my pain was coming from this source.

On July 12th, I was, once again, seeing my orthopedic physician. He told me *"this is a no choice situation now."* I needed a laminectomy, which meant removing the "roof" or complete backside of the L-4 vertebrae to relieve pressure on the spinal cord. He also believed that my hip, leg, and low back pain would be relieved, as well. Since the backside of my L-4 was to be removed, it was an opportunity to remove the soft tissue that was compressing the spinal cord, lift the spinal cord, and obtain a bone core biopsy of the now infamous "sweet spot" in my L-4 vertebrae. His main concern for the surgery was that the soft tissue and even the "sweet spot" within the L-4 vertebrae were hemangiomas—very bloody tumors (usually benign) that would bleed significantly during surgery.

I was more than a bit nervous about the surgery, and he went over the plastic model of the vertebrae with me. The L-4 vertebrae is a tough one to get at. The spinal cord splits into the leg nerves inside this vertebrae, and the femoral arteries and veins all split on the front side of this vertebrae. That is why surgery in and around this vertebrae is so difficult. The other thing that bothered me was that we were removing the only good piece of the vertebrae and "throwing it away." I asked what happens if the "bad" half had to be removed. My orthopedic physician said he had already discussed that possibility with colleagues. If that were to happen, I would also, at a later time, have to undergo the difficult frontal surgery to have the "bad" half removed, and struts would be made to span L-3 and L-5. I decided to take on one thing at a time.

I entered the hospital, in Denver, that was my orthopedic surgeon's favorite for surgery. This July 16th visit was for an outpatient procedure that was basically a search for the artery that was feeding the tumorous "mess" in my L-4 vertebrae. This was an angiogram and embolism procedure. The risky part of this procedure, in addition to a catheter inserted into the femoral artery, was the insertion of poly vinyl alcohol particles into the artery feeding the tumor, to block the blood flow to the capillary bed of the tumor. This was necessary prior to surgery for control of bleeding and to provide my surgeon's ability to see what he was doing.

When I was awakening from the procedure, the cardiac surgeon performing the angiogram said he could not find an artery. I asked:

"You could not find the artery?"

He replied, quite sternly: *"There isn't one to find!"*

I was not sure if this was his "ivory tower ego" speaking or if he was sure there was not one to find. The way my orthopedic physician had spoken, as well as the radiologists, I was under the assumption this was a sure thing. Now, it was questionable, in my mind, if this was a hemangioma. Medically, not finding an artery meant two things: first, it was probably not a hemangioma, and second, there was now less risk for the main surgery yet to come.

July 23rd was "major" surgery day. I checked in early, ready to move things ahead. The Medtronic pacemaker representative came to put my pacemaker into a "sleep" mode. There would be cauterization and monitors for which an electrical current may be running through my body and that could potentially damage the pacemaker.

The idea behind the surgery was two fold: First to relieve pressure coming from the soft tissue tumor around the spinal cord. Second, to get a biopsy from the "sweet spot" in L-4 that has been unreachable until now. The reason for not getting a biopsy sample from the front of L-4, as I previously stated, is the front of L-4 is hard to access as the vena cava and aorta cross at this point, and split off into the legs. Going in from the backside is an easier procedure but still challenging since the spinal cord begins to split into each of the legs. The process, in theory, is simple. The posterior or "roof" of L-4 is removed from the rest of the vertebrae. Unfortunately, this was the healthiest portion of my L-4 vertebrae, and it would be discarded. With the "roof" removed, the spinal cord would then be exposed, lifted from the remaining part of the vertebrae, and a bone core sample would be taken from the "sweet spot" to get the biopsy. While there, the soft tissue that was compressing the spinal cord was also removed for compression relief and a biopsy.

Since the spinal cord was compressed, my orthopedic physician's concern, in addition to potential bleeding, was the spinal cord would instantly push out and get "nicked" by the sawed bone edges not yet smoothed off. Part of the surgery team was, therefore, a "stitch person." This physician was specialized in quickly putting fine sutures into the spinal cord, as it was pushing its way out of the canal. I imagined the surgical suite looking like an old time boxing ring, with the fight manager, the "old stitch man," lots of towels draped over shoulders, and, of course, a "bell" between "rounds." I forgot to ask if and how many stitches were required, but it seems unimportant now.

On July 30th, the orthopedic physician called to say the results were in and it showed a low grade lymphoma. He also said I would probably get a little bit of radiation to take care of it. He is a positive and compassionate person and, I think, has a tough time giving bad news, so I had to ask for the details of exactly where the cancer was found. Cancer was found in the soft tissue that compressed the spinal cord, and was removed. Cancer was in the bone or the infamous "sweet spot," and cancer was also found in a lumbar disk.

Surgery was complete, and I was grateful to have a diagnosis. I needed a name for this so I could focus my energy—like I did in training for the Ironman® World Championship. I had no problem thinking positively. In fact, I did not want cancer, but since I knew I had it, I was excited to be on the next adventure. My orthopedic physician had discussed the findings with, and forwarded them to the oncologist.

I met, once again on August 6th, with the oncologist. He is a fairly young, very confident, and seemingly very verbally forceful. I got the impression that it was "his way or the highway." I was O.K. with that, however, as I wanted to attack cancer with swift force. In my past two meetings, when he was sure I did not have cancer, I felt he really did not want anything to do with me. Now, that I was a real patient, however, I think he had a sincere interest in my case. I had tremendous confidence in him, and I am convinced he was on "top of his game."

The first step was to "stage" my cancer. This was simply to make sure all the cancer was accounted for. He told me that there were many options for treatment, but we were probably talking about a combination of radiation and a "small bit of chemo." We had to check on a few things first, according to the oncologist: First, a bone marrow biopsy of each hip. Second, a lumbar tap. Third, CT scans with contrast. He said we could do the bone marrow biopsies and the lumbar tap right there, right then, in his office. He said he was the best at dong these and I would not need to be sedated. He was very, very wrong! The bone marrow biopsies were extremely painful, and to have it done without sedation is cruel and unusual punishment! The only thing interesting about the procedure was that he noted a significant difference in the feel of each hip. He decided not to do the lumbar tap, since he realized that my lower back anatomy was swollen and had changed significantly from my surgery. He decided to send me back to the hospital for a CT guided lumbar tap. Even though he said he was "the best" at doing a hip biopsy, afterwards he gave me an off-hand compliment: *"Gee, I've had Two hundred and fifty pound truck drivers that scream their heads off. You really took that well."* That was not a lot of consolation for the pain I endured.

I have had several myelograms and various other "lumbar pokes," but not with my back so sore from surgery, and the back of my hips still sore from the bone marrow biopsy. I showed up at the hospital on August 9th, very "squeamish" about getting another needle in my back and I decided I was going to ask for sedation. This interventional radiologist was sensitive to my condition; however sedation is not used in this procedure. Instead, he by—passed the surgical area, by about six inches above the "still tender" L-4 area, and inserted the needle in the L-2 area. This doctor and the nurse were very compassionate. They were very accommodating with their outright concern, compassion, and pleasant small talk. He was going to draw off 30cc's, but ended up with about twice that amount, or about ten percent of my spinal fluid. He said the lab would keep some for thirty days. If my oncologist needed any other kind of test on my spinal fluid—he'd have it without an additional procedure. This Doctor was thinking ahead for me and I appreciated it!

I was feeling very positive and "up," as this was the last of the difficult invasive tests. I kept thinking of the oncologist's words that *"this will be relatively easy to treat."*

I woke up on August 12th, having increasingly "weird" headaches since the last procedure, and I was concerned that I had a spinal leak. This is a bit of spinal fluid leaking out of the puncture into the spinal cord from last week's procedure. I called the hospital and spoke with one of the radiologists who concurred and thought it definitely sounded like a leak. They could "patch" it, which meant going back in to put a drop of my own blood on the puncture site, or I could try staying flat the rest of the day and night, and it might seal itself. To me, that sounded better than another "poke" in the back, so I drove home from work, stopping once to lie down, across the front seat, for a few minutes while my head "pounded."

August 16th, was a big day for me. I had a P.E.T. scan scheduled for that morning. This is the last of the diagnostic tests for staging, before treatment. I was very pleased about today. I felt it was a major milestone, as the next step is treatment and I really wanted to get on with it. Prior to a P.E.T. scan, I received an injection of nuclear tagged glucose. The idea is that cancer cells really "soak up" the sugar, so the P.E.T. would show any cancerous areas. A CT scan will show structure, and a P.E.T. scan will show activity. In other words, the metabolism of the cancer cells, processing sugar, will show up on a P.E.T. scan.

By August 19th, the staging was complete and I went to meet with the oncologist regarding the results and the treatment. While waiting for him, my wife, Mary Lou, asked me to explain all of the tests I had been undergoing, and how they related to the staging process. I explained that staging is like a golf score, but for cancer. The rating, for NHL (Non-Hodgkin's Lymphoma), is between I-IV, depending on how much the cancer is spread out in the body. The lower the score the better it is. If it is not spread out, it basically means that a targeted therapy, like radiation or surgery can be utilized. If it is a high score, it usually means a more "shot gun" or systemic therapy, like chemo therapy, needs to be utilized.

The oncologist came into the room and asked me what stage I thought I was at.

I replied: *"I think about a stage II, based on where I have felt the pain."* I asked what stage he thought I was at, before staging, and he replied:

"Well, remember I did not think you had cancer at all until the positive biopsy. I thought you would be a stage I."

"However," (what he told me next was surprising) *"The diagnostic tests show that you are well into stage IV, in fact, advanced stage IV—meaning we do not have options, we need to pull out the stops and treat with a full blown, six month course of chemotherapy, followed by some radiation."*

He again expressed his surprise that I did not look sick enough to be this "sick" with cancer! The diagnosis was made based on the P.E.T. scan, which showed cancer activity in the left humerus, the entire shaft of the right femur, and the L-4 vertebrae. No other diagnostic test indicated I had all that cancer. My first thought, honestly, was to wonder why we could not have started out with a P.E.T. scan. It would have saved the laminectomy of the L-4 vertebrae.

I TOLD THE ONCOLOGIST:

"I am very upbeat about all of this and I am really ready to move forward. But I have one question which I will ask one time and one time only: Why has it taken this long to be diagnosed?"

HIS REPLY WAS:

"I made a mistake, as did many other people." He said *"You have kept pathology departments in Denver and the Mayo Clinic in Mercedes Benz's for the last two years and everyone got it wrong."* Even though the oncologist did not give credit, I am grateful Dr. Carol, my "Coach" and endocrinologist, kept pushing for the right specialists to look at me, and evaluate my tests for the right answers. I also thought back to January, when this same oncologist said: *"there is no way you have cancer, you look too healthy."*

After that brief explanation of where I was at, it was a quick and easy shift to move things forward to treatment and a subsequent cure. The idea of "full blown chemotherapy" rattled me a bit, but now I had the full picture to deal with and focus on. I knew that the most effective way to move forward was not to dwell in the past. In addition, **nothing holds people from forward progress more that harboring anger about what was or what was not done in the past**. It was just "plain and simply" time to energize all my resources to move ahead.

August 21st was my day in "cancer school." Mary Lou and I were to get the whole scenario of what drugs, when and how they would be administered, side effects to expect, etc. from one of the cancer center nurses. I thought I under-stood and "got it" that this was going to be a serious treatment. I asked her about the probability of hair loss. The way the nurse looked at me and said, very clearly, *"one hundred percent within two weeks,"* I really "got it" that this was a serious treatment with very toxic drugs. I was going to receive eight courses of CHOP therapy, with the addition of a newer drug, Rituxan®, a monoclonal antibody. Rituxan® (rituximab) is a biological, while the other drugs are chemicals. The Chemicals in the CHOP acronom include: Cytoxin®(cyclophosphamide), Doxil® (doxorubicin), Oncovin® (vincristine), and prednisone. The first three, including Rituxan are administered via infusion, while the prednisone is oral. Since I was otherwise very healthy, the oncologist felt I could tolerate the sug-gested eight two day sessions in eight one day sessions.

My reaction to cancer was interesting. I wondered what I had done to deserve cancer! I was embarrassed to have cancer at first. It may have been, in part, from friends and family reactions to my diagnosis. Some were angry that I just now received a serious diagnosis after having a wrong diagnosis for so long. Others that I rarely spoke with came out of the woodwork to lend support. Some wanted to tell me about their aches and pains. The most humorous were the many kind hearted folks who looked over both shoulders before whispering something like: *"my uncle's best friend has a cousin who had cancer cured by a tea you can only buy in Mexico. I'll be glad to find out what it was for you."*

On August 23rd, I went to the "back surgery" hospital for a nuclear bone scan. This is the same type of test I had a year ago that identified all of the "hot spots," where I had bone activity which was thought to be Paget's Disease. This scan actually shows any bone activity. For example, it would show a hair line stress fracture that does not show up on an X-ray. In this example, the scan does not permit the physician to say "this is a tiny stress fracture." It merely indicates bone activity of some type that may indicate a tiny stress facture or some other "abnormality"

The nuclear bone scan is much less expensive than a P.E.T. Scan, and since my P.E.T. scan results showing cancer was basically a mirror image of the bone activity of my nuclear bone scan, the simple and relatively inexpensive nuclear bone scan would be used to determine efficacy and progress of my chemotherapy.

After receiving the injection of nuclear material, I had two hours to "kill" and drink water. I went over to the University to check out the classroom that was assigned for my class.

4

My Second Ironman® Event

Time Line: 2001: February, March, April, May, June, July, August, September, October, November, December
Time Line: 2002: January, February, March, April, May, June, July, August, September

Principle 7: Do Not Ask Why Me?—Ask Why Not Me?

I confess, I did ask myself, a few times "why me?" How could I have cancer? Since my first Ironman® World Championship, I have eaten very healthy, I have maintained a well above average exercise level, I have never, smoked, etc. My biggest fitness "sin" was an occasional Snickers® bar. After twenty-some years, I was still an invincible Ironman®—and then I thought—"why not me?" I can do this. I proved myself in the "original" Ironman® World Championship twenty years ago—and this was going to be my second Ironman®—only without the swimming, biking, and running.

Asking "why not me" and believing I could do this was the first step—just like in my first Ironman® World Championship in Kona, Hawaii. Second, I pictured myself at the end of treatment—healthy, cancer free, and feeling good. Once I pictured myself at "the finish line," I turned to see what "stepping stones" there where to help achieve my goal. Since I had no obstacles—only "stepping stones," I would never have to "fight" cancer. I did not "fight" to finish the Ironman® World Championship. I enjoyed every bit of the training and the event. I was going to take on this "second" Ironman® race with the same positive attitude, learn all I could, stay in the best physical condition during treatment, and accomplish my goals. Even spiritually, I never prayed, asking for a cure—I prayed to give thanks for the adventurous healing process.

I was anxious to get ready for my "second" Ironman® race. I purchased all of the supplies I learned I would need from my "cancer school" session. I purchased Senakot® for constipation, Imodium® for diarrhea, and Ensure® for nutrition. I never thought I would ever be buying these things, but I accepted it as part of the adventure.

I also bought what seemed like a lifetime supply of Lysol® disinfectant spray, disinfectant wipes, and a gallon of liquid Dial® soap. The "make or break" of this therapy as I learned, is to stay clear of any infections, as the chemotherapy would lower the white cell count, and thus the body's ability to fight off infections.

The second "make or break" issue is nutrition. I tasted one of the cans of Ensure®. The taste brought back a lot of memories of my first Ironman® World Championship training, as I drank three cans of Nutriment® (a very similar product) while training in 1982. Twenty years later, I feel very similar to how I felt during the "original" Ironman® World Championship. I wrote in my journal: *"I am so ready for this event!"*

I also decided to cut my hair short, since I was going to lose it soon. I surprised myself for my greatest Ironman® event to go one step further by asking a hair stylist to "buzz" my head and then shave lightening bolts into each side of my scalp. I was going into this Ironman® with unstoppable attitude!

There was a very interesting sermon in church, August 25. The topic was the importance in living now. The sermon was about a friend of the pastor that was miss-diagnosed for seven months. He was finally diagnosed with lymphoma cancer in his bones. He was successfully treated, only to have a fast relapse and then "passed on." The story was hauntingly similar, at least the first part. I had already pictured my successful completion of chemotherapy, and a relapse and death were not in that picture. I left that church service somewhat stunned by the rare similarity of a diagnosis problem and even further by a rare occurrence of lymphoma in the bones.

I was awake early, as I often had been in the course of this year. Whether by pain or insomnia, 1:30am no longer seemed like an abnormal hour to wake up and get up. Mary Lou and I showed up at the cancer center at 9am, August 28th. I was introduced to what would be a routine ritual for some time to come. First, there was a quick check of the vital signs, which includes temperature, weight, and blood pressure. Blood was also taken to run all of the necessary lab tests, the most important being the white cell count. My white cell count, as the tests determined, was already on the low side.

In most cancer centers, the patients can sit in chairs arranged in a "social" setting, and in some centers, there are optional rooms where a patient can receive the treatment alone, or have privacy with a family member. I opted for the private room. I had investigated some patient support groups for Paget's, and decided I did not want to "hang around" with people thinking of themselves as sick. Now I realize cancer patients, in general, are very positive people!

I had a case of *"Unstoppable Attitude,"* and I had cancer. I was not sick!

It was a humbling experience to be getting chemotherapy. It was not just the chemotherapy drugs I was going to be receiving. There was Benadryl® for possible allergic reactions, an antinauseant, a steroid, and an analgesic. Three of the chemotherapy drugs were from companies I had worked for or consulted with in the past. While I was not involved with the anticancer drugs when I worked with these companies, I was aware of their toxicity. In fact, one was called "red poison" by the manufacturing group that made it. (The same drug was called "red gold" by the finance department.) My vital signs were monitored closely on this first visit. The complete process took about eight hours. That long period of time and the toxicity of those drugs "drove home" the seriousness of these treatments and the cancer we were going to win against.

I was drowsy and dosed off and on much of the time during the afternoon of the chemotherapy session. We needed to stop at the store on the way home to pick up some Compazine®, as they forgot to tell us, at "chemo school" to get some for nausea. About an hour after I got home, I felt like a truck had hit me (yes, I do know, as I have been hit once by a pickup truck, while riding my bicycle). I started to feel better as the evening progressed, and finally slept for about four hours. I stayed home from work the next day and slept for about three hours each in the morning and afternoon.

I woke up about two am, August 31st, and by five am, I was clutching a garbage can. I was quite frightened as I did not know if this was the start of a continuous "sick" six months. I would have seven more sessions of chemotherapy during the next six months. My "stepping stones" were to continue to work at my day job, teach my one class per semester at the University of Colorado on Tuesday nights, and stay as healthy as I could through nutrition, exercise, and extreme cleanliness to stay free from infections. I remembered saying to myself: *"this is not an obstacle—only a stepping stone! It will get me to tomorrow and the next day, and I'll feel better!"*

It was September 8th and I happened to look into a mirror. For the first time, probably since my first Ironman® World Championship in 1982, I saw cheek bones in my face. I was amazed at how tired and run down I had become in such a short time after my first chemotherapy session. I now had many questions after this session: Will this get worse? Will I tolerate the side effects better? What can I do to make this better? On a lighter side, this was day eleven after my first chemotherapy session. I was supposed to lose my hair sometime between day ten and day fourteen. Everything seemed pretty well anchored in my body. I actually had visions of being an Ironman® "too tough" to lose my hair.

I was having trouble getting significant sleep. Much of the cause, I believe was the prednisone I took as part of the chemotherapy regimen. This caught up relatively fast, as I worked all day and taught class Tuesday nights, not getting home until 10:00pm. I think it took a few days to recover, but the tiredness, combined with my thin face, "so soon" had me a bit concerned. I thought I may have started this race too fast, outpacing myself too soon.

My thoughts went back to my running experience. I did the same in the New York Marathon in 1981. I had not trained enough because of a broken foot I suffered in my first marathon six months prior. I had stress fractures from over training. I started the New York marathon with much "foot healing time", but very little training. At the ten mile mark, my time was sixty minutes flat. I felt good, even at this six minute mile pace, but I knew I started the race too fast, and could be in serious trouble later in the race—and I was!

I went in for my second chemotherapy session on September 18th. Unfortunately, my white cell count was too low to receive treatment. The oncologist said it would probably be high enough after the weekend, on Monday. He also said that if I was up for it, I could come in two days later on Friday morning for a blood test, and if it was O.K., I could receive treatment then. I was in this Ironman® race to finish, and finish well, including the time. Therefore, I "showed up" and went in Friday morning, passed the blood test and received the second round of chemotherapy.

In addition to noticing continual changes in my face, I lost all of my hair before my 3rd chemo session. Driving home from work, one day, I scratched my head and noticed a tuft of hair came out. I opened the car window, as I drove, stuck my head out, and began pulling out much of my hair. I found this to be an amusing experience, spreading my hair over a thirty mile stretch of highway! Losing my hair was no big deal. I can understand, although, why to many women, this can be a disturbing side effect. For men, however, I don't understand why it is bothersome. For me, particularly when the lightening bolts that were shaved into my scalp had tanned and remained visible for quite some time, baldness was a minor part of the adventure!

Over the six months of therapy, each of the eight chemotherapy sessions became similar. Each evening, I had that "hit by a truck" feeling. I would have difficulty sleeping over the next two weeks. I would have an increasing adrenaline rush from my growing, unstoppable attitude. I was less and less sick, although the entire six months were similar to living with a bad case of the flu and feeling all of the flu-like symptoms of feeling tired, sick, and achy all over.

As treatment progressed, I was instructed to give myself a shot of Neulasta®, a white cell protein stimulator, a day after each of my chemotherapy sessions. When I first discussed Neulasta® with the nurse, she trained me how to self inject into my thigh. I did not think it would be a "tough thing" to do, however once during a chemotherapy session, a woman was to receive the same shot in her arm. As she was about to "get it," she turned away from the nurse who was administering the shot, and towards me, as she made a "painfully gut wrenching" face. This "set me up," and the first time I thrust the needle into my leg, required a bit of courage! Again, this was not an obstacle. This was another "stepping stone." It worked very well, and the oncologist was very surprised with the efficacy it had in my body.

I also maintained a minimal amount of exercise, now in the form of walking. Unfortunately, I was unable to swim due to the risk of infection from pool water. I walked every day. I worked, taught classes for the SBA, coached entrepreneurs and taught my Tuesday night graduate class at the University Of Colorado Denver. There was always someone from the Community College ready to take a walk with me. I later realized how much everyone there kept an eye out for my well being and I really appreciate all the benefits I received from such concern.

My University MBA marketing class had an interesting "ring side" seat to my race. The first class meeting of the semester was the night before my first chemotherapy. I had a bit of trouble getting out my message to the class, that night, but I basically told them the following:

"You can't live life from a vacuum and you can't market from a vacuum, and I do not teach marketing from a vacuum. In the real world things happen that you need to react to, change strategies for, and generally, be aware that changes are part of the "norm." You will see some changes in this class, particularly with me. I start chemotherapy tomorrow. I expect to be here every Tuesday night. You will see me go through physical changes such as hair and weight loss. I have already pictured, in my mind, completing all of my chemotherapy sessions, continuing to teach this class, and beating cancer. This is a done deal! All I need to do is to handle all of the things that ensure my vision of success. So every assignment in class will be via Email. If you have a cold

or are feeling sick—please sit towards the back of the room. Please do not step beyond the edge of the instructor's desk when approaching.

Principle 8: Inspire Others To, In Turn, Inspire Others

I prepared for each class in the same way. I pulled out a can of Lysol™ spray, and disinfectant wipes and completely cleaned off the desk, and all of the electronic gear I would be using. As I did this, several class members would walk in and "take stock" in how my looks changed from the week before. Many would ask how I was doing, or simply give me a "thumbs up." The most incredibly rewarding evening was the last. A student approached me and said his wife alerted him to the fact that this was the first class in his entire college career that he never missed "even one" class session. This perfect attendance record was something he never accomplished, even in undergraduate school. He told me he really liked the class and would have shown up anyway. However, he would not dare miss a class, *"knowing that the professor was not going to miss a class, even with what he was going through."* I had inspired someone, and felt a great sense of Ironman® accomplishment. I have often said one of the best things in life is to inspire someone. The ultimate is to inspire someone to, in turn, inspire others. His inspiration inspired me. Right then "my world was a perfect place."

The most difficult period of the six month cancer treatment was the midway point. I had completed four sessions, and had four left to go. It was similar to a bicycle ride up a long hill, anticipating the downhill ride on the other side, but finding out you had to ride a slow ten miles across a flat plateau. The three weeks in between dragged on forever. I had no control over moving things forward. All I could do was cross the plateau and think about the exhilarating downhill finish of this "chemo" Ironman® race.

Every other week I had an especially tiring schedule at work. On Monday, I taught a small business class at 7:30am at the community college, where my office was. On Wednesday, I taught a noon small business class at a different community college campus about 25 miles away, and on Thursday, I taught an evening small business class at yet another community college campus, and then drove about fifty miles home. During the day, I saw small business clients in my office, and, of course, on Tuesday nights I taught the marketing class at the University. I constantly ran on adrenalin, similar to training for and being in the Ironman® World Championship. I kept as busy as I could, staying in the "race." The whole time, I never lost sight of my cancer free goals, and never eased up on the things that were necessary to ensure accomplishing those goals.

In September Dr. Carol was going to present "my case" to the Metabolic Bone Disease Society of Colorado to about one hundred physicians. She had also discussed "my case" with several national experts at an earlier meeting in Texas. Having worked in the pharmaceutical and biotechnology industry, I had attended many medical meetings and presentations—but never as a patient. I was very pleased when she invited me to attend the meeting. This was another difference that made Dr. Carol stand above the "ordinary." My oncologist once told me he was presenting "my case" to a small group of oncologists. I suggested I attend the meeting, since one of the continuing difficulties of "my case" was that my physical appearance did not indicate the underlying disease or its severity. He was somewhat "stunned" that I suggested it, and replied that "these doctors are not really used to seeing actual patients." By now, I am convinced that they should be!

Dr. Carol, on the other hand, had a very patient oriented attitude. I would even call it "Unstoppable Attitude." She even asked me to review the slides for dates of procedures, and background information. I was pleased to do so. She did a great job organizing and delivering the presentation. It was presented in the chronological order that "my case" unfolded. She had a radiologist read the X-rays, and CT scans, as they were read and reported on by the radiologists during my long time diagnosis.

The presentation was somewhat of a turning point for me. While I was not dwelling in the past, only the successful completion of this Ironman® race, her presentation provided me with much insight as to why things seemed to drag on to get my final diagnosis. Dr. Carol suggested I sit in the back of the room, and she would introduce me to the audience at the end of the presentation, as I was "hairless" and obviously on chemotherapy. Her presentation was interactive, and the physician audience was taken through the case and asked to "vote" on their next options. So, for them to see me, bald and pale, would obviously give away the final cancer diagnosis.

By mistake, the physician moderator of the program introduced me before the presentation, so I stood and gave a wave to the audience. For sure, I thought, the cancer diagnosis was a "dead" give away. However, Dr. Carol went on and presented my case step by step, with the X-rays, CT scans, and lab results, just as they happened and as they were presented to my team of physicians. At the end of the presentation, the diagnosis of cancer was not chosen by the group, even after seeing me in my obvious cancer treatment state! At that point I realized that mine really was a "tough case" to diagnose.

One thing the group did agree on later, however, was my osteoporosis was most probably caused by my cancer, and they agreed I should be treated with Aredia infusions. There were some very surprised expressions when the audience was told the actual NHL cancer diagnosis, many physicians turned around and gave me a second look. The highlights of reviewing "my case" were; the difficulty in diagnosing, the difficulty in determining what type of lymphoma cancer I had (and I still do not have a complete identification), and for the first time cancer was identified as a cause of osteoporosis. The latter was based on the fact I have always been so active; there was no other reason to have osteoporosis. I hoped that this information, as well as my entire case would help someone, somehow, someday!

Still running on adrenaline, which could be the "chemical" name for *"Unstoppable Attitude,"* I kept up with my schedule of work and teaching, exercising, nutrition, and hygiene. Just like my first Ironman® World Championship, when I had mentally finished the race one year before I ran it, I was already mentally cured of cancer. It was a "done deal." I was mentally "there" at the finish line, and had been for six months. It was always just a matter of mentally looking back from the finish line and figuring out how I got there. It was staying busy, keeping fueled with proper nutrition, exercising, keeping a high degree of hygiene, and living my *"Unstoppable Attitude."* Even spiritually, I never prayed to ask for a cure—I prayed to give thanks for the adventurous healing.

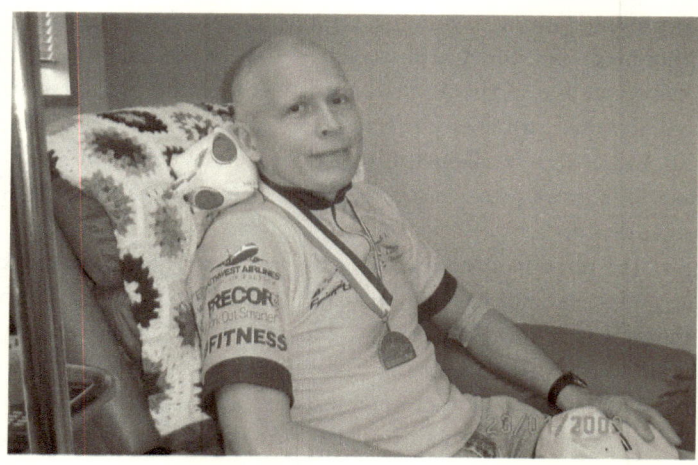

My "look" for most of my Ironman® cancer race

Nutrition was somewhat difficult during the six months. The Ensure® that tasted so good prior to the start of chemotherapy was "unthinkable" within two days after I started. Basically every food I liked prior to chemotherapy was the first to turn me "green" at the slightest thought of them. Unfortunately water was the most difficult. Hydration was important during chemotherapy, just as it was a key component in the lava fields of Hawaii during my first Ironman® World Championship. Now, water tasted how I imagine "Three In One™" oil tasted. I had to constantly figure out ways to flavor my water.

I progressively tolerated the effects of chemotherapy better during the six months. I had less nausea with each treatment, but continually felt like I had a "nasty" case of the flu. By the end of the third week, after each chemotherapy session, I started to feel somewhat normal. I then knew it was time for another session in the next couple of days. I was able to actually ride my bicycle a couple of times for twenty miles, up in the mountains. I was still having pain, however, not as bad as before. I was aware of the right femur, right hip, and tailbone soreness. I attributed it to cancer cells being killed.

I had many "stand out" moments during my chemotherapy. The "biggest" was in October when I received an autograph yellow bicycle jersey from the Northern California Chapter of Team In Training®. Susan, a friend of mine, whom I worked with for a short time, had been interested in triathlons. She enthusiastically jumped into the sport. After awhile, she became interested in Team in Training®, the sporting organization that raises a tremendous amount of money for Lymphoma cancer research. When she learned I was being treated for Paget's, she "unofficially" sponsored me by carrying my name on her bicycle during their group rides. I explained I did not have cancer, but she knew I was having a challenge and she wanted to keep me in mind during her rides. Well, a year later, I was finally diagnosed with Lymphoma cancer, and she now legitimately carried my name on her bike. In fact, I was now sponsored by the entire team. I was tremendously moved to receive the yellow jersey of the Northern California Chapter that was autographed with well wishes from all of the team members. I decided I was going to wear this jersey and my Ironman® World Championship medal on the day of my last chemo therapy, the finish line to my "second" Ironman® Cancer Championship.

There were many "little" things that had large impacts on me during the six months of treatment. As each treatment session progressed, it became more and more difficult for the nurses to "hit" a vein to start an IV. My veins started to take on a hardness and "evasive" quality when it came time for the needle. So often it was taking up to four attempts to get the IV going, and that was four attempts with each one consisting of sticking, wiggling, and poking several times. So on my fourth chemotherapy session, I was delighted that the oncology "nurse for the day" hit the vein on her first try. In addition, she did not like to use the IV Pump that regulated the flow of chemicals. Instead, she ran the chemicals through directly and a bit faster and monitored the vital signs to make sure everything was O.K. It was nice to complete the fourth session in about six hours.

Another "little" thing was finding out I could take my dose of prednisone on the morning after each chemotherapy session, as opposed to the evening of the same day. No wonder I was sick and unable to sleep. Just that simple switch to the "morning after" helped a tremendous amount in getting my sleep requirement. The oral prednisone was one of the "small but challenging" ingredients of the drug regimen. The taste is so terrible; the five tablets could not be swallowed fast enough. Prednisone leaves one "wired." Taking that amount at night virtually guaranteed a night of little sleep. The term I started using for my trouble sleeping was "rotisserie sleeping," as I just kept turning over and over.

I made an appointment with my orthopedic surgeon to have my femur X-rayed and checked out. He thought I was still in the "little bit of cancer" and "easy to treat" mode. He was very surprised to see me hairless, and being treated for stage IV bone cancer. He X-rayed the femur and told me that if it got any worse, I might need to have a stainless steel rod inserted in the bone to keep it from breaking. I immediately thought that if my femur was that weak, I would sooner opt for a "piece of wood and duct tape," and I did not hesitate in telling him so!

Mary Lou and I took a road trip to Las Vegas for Thanksgiving. We were both ready to break the cycle of work, chemo, and work. Greg was going to school in Las Vegas, and Kelly flew in from Boston. It was the first time they both saw me without hair. Interestingly, I had eyebrows when I arrived in Vegas, but had none when I left. (What my eyebrows did in Vegas—they stayed in Vegas!) I was truly hairless. Also, it was the third week after my fifth chemotherapy session, and I was feeling pretty good. We ate at a buffet, and I was surprised to find enough things to eat at the buffet to be very full! As uplifting as the trip was, it was very tiring. While I felt a bit less sick with each chemotherapy session, I was getting more and more tired.

When December came, I could see the light at the end of the tunnel. I had three more chemotherapy sessions to complete over a two month period and I was looking forward to putting on the yellow jersey. By the end of January, I would be done! I had a bone scan done on November 19th, for a "half way" look at the "standings." I did not get the results, from one of the oncology nurses until

December 3rd, after several calls. The bone scan was to indicate progress because it was thought it correlated with the more expensive P.E.T. Scan. The scan showed a persistent no change "uptake" of nuclear material in the right femur, two new areas of uptake in each mid tibial shafts, and a mild increase in the midline in the lower neck. I had some questions for the oncologist, but for now, I was heading for the finish line and I put a positive "spin" on the report for Mary Lou. I realized that my being positive not only keeps everyone else positive, but it works to keep myself positive as well. I knew I was winning this Ironman® race. It is a "done deal" that I wanted to be over.

On January 23rd, 2003, I received my last chemotherapy session. For the event, I wore the autographed yellow jersey, sent from the Northern California Chapter of Team in Training. I also took my old Ironman® medal from 1982 "out of retirement" for this "second" Ironman® finish. Like the first Ironman®, I had accomplished my goals. Crossing the finish line was a celebration of accomplishing those goals.

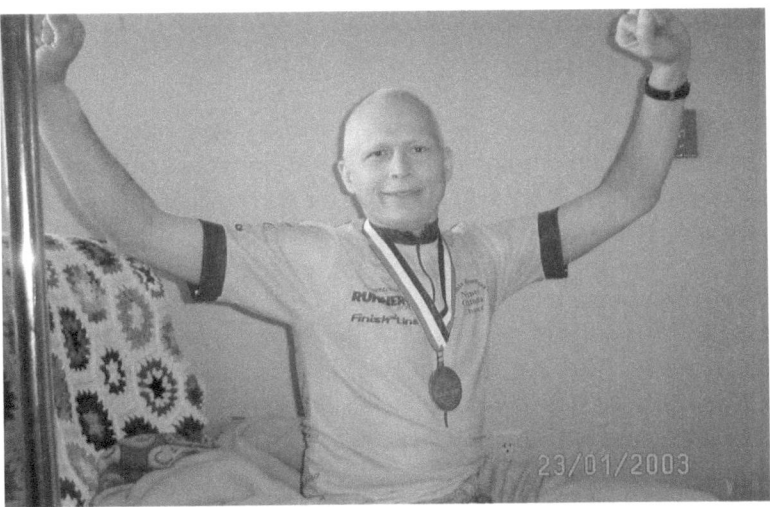

Crossing the finish line of my first Ironman® Cancer Championship!

5

Remission

Principle 9: Surround Yourself With Positive, Supporting People

I was fortunate to have taken the position with a community college environment. Front Range Community College in Westminster was my healthy environment for working while I was being treated for cancer. The college was a wealth of positive and supporting people. Linda, whom I worked with closely, not only assisted me in work matters, she excelled in keeping a sense of humor about so many things. I attribute many healing laughs from her compassionate, humerus, *"Unstoppable Attitude!"* My experience at the college was highlighted when Bill Richards, then Vice President, asked if I would deliver the spring commencement address. He explained how everyone was so proud to have watched me conquer my cancer with such an *"Unstoppable Attitude."*

With humble honor, and a very high level energy, I took on this challenge, and in April, delivered the commencement address to an audience of over 1200 graduates and their family members. I was so proud to have my Front Range Community college colleagues proud of me! This wonderful event also marked the first time I described my ten principles of "Unstoppable Attitude" to anyone. Since then, I knew it was important to share them.

To me, the commencement address was a "time to move on signal." It is not that I wanted to put distance between my life and cancer. I just wanted to move on. In February, 2003, I had the "re-staging" done to show the cancer was gone.

The CT scan was O.K., as it always had been. The P.E.T. scan report, however, indicated a small area of activity in the L-4 vertebrae.

My oncologist said it was the *"radiologist that was covering his rear,"* and that the amount of activity was within normal limits. In addition, he added, the chemotherapy was still in my system working. He went out of the room to phone the radiologist, and I heard him, just outside the exam room, verbally "beat up" the radiologist into changing the report. The next day, I had a new P.E.T. scan report that said I was "clear." I asked my oncologist if this meant I was now in remission. He said, "yes, absolutely." I walked away feeling this was a bit of a "wishy washy" confirmation of remission, but I took it!

I submitted my findings to Dr. Carol, who agreed there were a number of "loose ends" in my case, and sent me and my records to the University of Colorado Oncology department. The University Oncologist said the best thing to do was probably wait for the six month check. I was having an increase in "tail bone" pain, and waking most nights around 2:00am with pain in my right femur and the neuropathy in my left leg.

In April, I was asked to write and conduct a sales training course for a biotechnology company in Boulder. I was ready to get back to the "real world" with what I thought was a "real world" paycheck, so I volunteered my time and donated the money back to the college. I started the two day training in early May, and quickly realized the company had a lot of potential, at least in generating sales. Although I was not all that familiar with the product line, synthetic DNA, (ironically much used for cancer research), I was convinced they were not targeting the right markets.

I was asked to interview for the director of marketing position they had open. Prior to the interview, I learned they were also looking for a General Manager. I decided that position was to be mine, and during the interview for the marketing director, I told them I was not interested, as I had "been there, done that." So I positioned myself for the GM spot, and won it. I told both the CEO, and my future boss *"I am the guy that can take this division to number one in the market".* The corporate CEO laughed—at first, but then realized how serious I was.

I now had a team of young adults for which I had the responsibility to inspire, I took that responsibility very seriously. Many of them had Ph.D.s in chemistry and biochemistry. They were smarter than me, and when they began to feel the power of *"Unstoppable Attitude,"* the "DNA Factory" as we began to affectionately call the division, began to gain forward momentum. In one year, our sales and corresponding level of success went from $1 million to $6 million. What changed to make such a drastic change?

Authentic, "Unstoppable Attitude!"

Cancer was now in my past, and I was totally into the business, with the stress, long hours, and a difficult learning curve for the biotechnology business the company was focused on. I started walking for exercise, and was feeling pretty good. So when my six month check up time approached, I was aware of "needing" the CT scan and P.E.T. scan, and was aware my oncologist had not contacted me for these tests. I found myself getting a bit angry about his lack of initiative in contacting me, and at the same time, I was a bit reluctant to get the test results. I started calling his office to get them to schedule the test, and after several calls, the tests were scheduled. I called my oncologist several times in the next two weeks. I knew the report was available, but he just did not call back.

Feeling very frustrated, I asked his nurse what was going on, and she said she did not know why he was not returning a call to me. I asked her to read me the report, and she did. Once again the P.E.T. Scan showed an increase in uptake activity in the L-4 vertebrae. When I finally spoke with the oncologist after three weeks, his response was:

"I did not know what to tell you, so I have not called."

He suggested, again that the radiologists were too far on the cautious side, but we could repeat the tests in two months. I again sought a second opinion from the University of Colorado Health Science Center oncologists, on November 3. Again, they said that the prudent thing would be to redo the tests in a couple of months. At this time, the chief oncologist said he was now suspecting a "fast moving, aggressive" cancer. Originally, my oncologist had said that it was a slow moving cancer that I may have had for several years. The next set of P.E.T. scans, two months later, showed an even greater activity of cancer, and now there was no question this was a fast moving cancer. Structurally, it appeared to be a slow growing cancer type. Metabolically, however, it was growing very fast.

6

My "Third" Ironman® Race Begins

Time Line: 2001: February, March, April, May, June, July, August, September, October, November, December
Time Line: 2002: January, February, March, April, May, June, July, August, September, October, November, December
Time Line: 2003: January, February, March, April, May, June, July, August, September, October, November

The problem, however, was that no one was going to treat me for a recurring cancer without a positive biopsy. I was scheduled, once again, for a bone core biopsy of L-4 at the hospital where I had my first core biopsy. I checked in for the procedure on December 31, 2003, was prepped, hooked up to an I.V. line and ready to go, when a nurse came in the room and told me the interventional radiologist was not going to do the procedure. She removed the I.V. line, and told me to get dressed, and she would take me to the X-Ray reading room, as the Doctor wanted to speak with me.

When I entered, the Radiologist was looking at a wall of films on light boxes, the majority of which were mine. Two other physicians were looking at my films. He introduced himself and the others to me, and started showing me what their conclusions were. They were quite sure of two things: First, the "spot" that needed to have a biopsy was almost impossible to get at. Second, the area in the vertebrae that contained the "spot" appeared to be a hemangioma. I surprised them when I discussed my case history of the physicians' first thinking this was a hemangioma, and getting a negative angiogram to find an artery feeding the "alleged" hemangioma. I showed them where my orthopedic physician had taken a core sample from underneath the spinal cord. We had a very good discussion, and I was feeling good and somewhat surprised that I was able to verbalize, with fairly good medical detail, what my case was all about, and used some of the scans to do so. The main Interventional radiologist asked me what the next step was if they did not do the core biopsy. I replied that no one was going to treat this "pretty obvious" cancer unless they received a confirmation by a positive biopsy.

I said: *"If we cannot do a core biopsy here today, I will need to undergo major surgery to get a biopsy through my front side."*

Again, the radiologists all looked at me and discussed how difficult it would be to get a sample from the "sweet spot."

One radiologist asked: *"What happens if we get a sample, and it is negative?"*

I replied, *"If I do not get a positive core sample, I will still need the surgery."*

They agreed the surgery would be pretty drastic, and the main interventional radiologist said, with a great amount of sincerity:

"I will do everything I can to get a sample from that area."

It seems a bit strange, that someone would want a biopsy that was positive for cancer. I knew, and so did most of my doctors that I had cancer. The open surgery to confirm what we all knew was going to be drastic, and leave me in a pretty weak state to treat cancer, once again. The nurses were surprised to see me stroll back to the pre-op room and ask them to re-prep me, complete with I.V., for the procedure. Like the other bone core sample procedures, I was "foggily" aware of some of the tugging during the procedure, and I remember several people in the room, probably extra radiologists, and a couple of pathologists.

I owe a lot to that interventional radiologist. He did the "almost impossible" and got a core sample from the "sweet spot." In the first week of January 2004, I, once again, had a diagnosis of a lymphoma cancer in the L-4 vertebrae. On my visit to my oncologist, he said:

"It was a lymphoma type that "should not be in the bone, without first being in soft tissue, some where, and it looks like a "low grade" lymphoma that should not be acting aggressively, but that's what we have, and you need to speak with the bone marrow transplant "guys" downtown."

On January 12th, 2004, I had my first appointment with the transplant "team." I had started to investigate the process on the internet, but was totally unprepared for the magnitude of this process. If my first cancer treatment was a boxing match, this was going to be the world heavy weight event. If my first cancer treatment was a bicycle race, this was going to be the Tour de France. If my first cancer treatment was a marathon, this was going to be the Ironman® World Championship. As such, this professional group was appropriately highly trained, and I "got it"—I *really* "got it" that I would be treated, both myself and my cancer, in a highly professional and supportive manner. My transplant physician had recently joined the group from the University, so he was aware of my case from my primary oncologist, as well as the university oncologist from whom I received my second opinion from. The nursing staff, insurance staff, scheduling staff, etc.,—all were "top", "A-1" professionals.

When my new transplant physician suggested I would be getting my pre-treatment chemo from my primary oncologist who treated my first cancer, I declined. I then called his office and told his staff that I would be receiving my treatment "down town" at the Bone Marrow Transplant (BMT) Center, because of a change in my geographic location. It made more sense to be driving down town for treatment, instead of the northern suburb office where I was treated the year before. Essentially, however, what I was really delivering, to my first oncologist, was a now popular Donald Trump-ism, "you're fired."

My first bone marrow biopsy was scheduled for January 21st. This was the procedure that was done by my first oncologist, in his office, without sedation. The nurse practitioners were "jolted" when I told them of my previous experience, and they assured me they would be sedating me—and they did! This major procedure, which had kept me up at night worrying because of my first experience, was a "piece of cake." My initial confidence and good feeling about the Bone Marrow Transplant center was solidified from this experience. Two days after the biopsy, I was snowboarding with little discomfort—the true test of a bone marrow biopsy well performed. The results of the bone marrow biopsy were good. Not much more than the normal amount of cancer cells, which made the possibility of using my own stem cells for the transplant a good possibility.

On January 24th, Dr. Carol called to wish me well, and assured me that she would bring my new bone marrow transplant oncologists up to speed on my bone condition, and instructions to administer the Aredia®. When you win big once, with a great coach, it is great to have that coach there for the next event.

The bone marrow transplant (BMT) process is, to say the least, is an amazing procedure. There are two main types of bone marrow transplant: In an allogeneic transplant, another person's bone marrow cells are used to restore bone marrow after high dose chemotherapy and sometimes radiation therapy. In some cases, patients may be their own bone marrow donors. I am one of these, and I had an autologous BMT.

Bone marrow is the soft, spongy tissue found inside bones. The bone marrow in the breast bone, skull, hips, ribs and spine contains stem cells that produce the body's blood cells. These blood cells include white blood cells (leukocytes), which fight infection; red blood cells (erythrocytes), which carry oxygen to, and remove waste products from organs and tissues; and platelets, which enable the blood to clot.

Basically, in the case of my cancer, I had cancer cells that overcame the treatment results of my first cancer. Since it was all happening in the bone, there was a potential of the cancer cells being spread, by the blood stream, to other organs. Large doses of toxic chemotherapy were required to destroy the abnormal cancer cells. These treatments, however, not only kill the abnormal cells but destroy normal cells found in the bone marrow as well as soft tissue. That is what makes the BMT process tough. A bone marrow transplant enabled physicians to treat my cancer with aggressive chemotherapy by allowing replacement (using my own collected stem cells) of the diseased or damaged bone marrow that was left following the high dose chemotherapy.

Preparing For the Transplant

Time Line: 2001: February, March, April, May, June, July, August, September, October, November, December
Time Line: 2002: January, February, March, April, May, June, July, August, September, October, November, December
Time Line: 2003: January, February, March, April, May, June, July, August, September, October, November, December
Time Line: 2004: January

Preparing for a bone marrow transplant can be daunting. There are major finance and/or insurance issues, time off work issues, and family issues. The more one can learn of the process, and what is involved, the better off one is to take this race on. This was going to be my "third Ironman® race," and it was going to be the biggest, with the furthest "distance" to reach the finish line. On January 28, 2004, I had my PIC line put in at the hospital. The PIC (percutaneous intravenous catheter) is an easy access to draw blood and administer drugs and chemotherapy. It is a line that was inserted into my right arm, inside and below the bicep. Two ports were left to "dangle" and the catheter itself extended into a venous pool near the heart. Towards the middle of the CHOP-R therapy, the previous year, my veins had become "chemo veins"—they refused to have a needle stuck into them without a good fight. It was often taking several attempts to finally get an IV going. So, for this round, the idea of a "long term" IV was fairly easy to accept.

Mary Lou took over the responsibility of "line maintenance" for these, and a bigger one, in my chest, yet to come. Every morning, the kitchen "center island" was thoroughly cleaned and disinfected. Heparin was drawn from a vial into a syringe, which she then used to "flush" the lines. It was a daily reminder that this was serious "race," and I was to stay focused on the positive outcome.

My recollection of the entire bone marrow transplant procedure is very "foggy," since the pre-transplant preparation chemotherapy was stronger than my previous CHOP + R. The fogginess can be illustrated best by an early amusing experience. While driving into the BMT center, one morning, Mary Lou asked if I wanted to stop for coffee and doughnuts. I looked at her and asked if she was kidding? The thought of a doughnut sounded completely terrible and made me feel sick.

She said: *"Well since you had one yesterday, I thought you might want one today."*

I could not believe what she was saying: *"No Way! Why would I do such an awful sounding thing? I'd be sick before I'd get to the door."*

Mary Lou kept insisting that we had stopped the day before, because I was so insistence that we had not made that stop, and she suggested I may have the receipt in my wallet. I did! In fact, I had two doughnuts and coffee!!!

The pre transplant chemotherapy was tough, but I was focused on crossing the finish line of my "third" Ironman® race. I was starting to take a few days off from work for my chemo therapy sessions. I also persuaded Mary Lou to drive us to Keystone Resort, once in a while to snowboard. Several of those times, it was for only one very slow, easy ride down the easiest slope, and a couple of times it was a chairlift ride up to catch a view, and a chairlift ride back down.

There were a few major side effects from this treatment. One day my balance was "knocked" out, and in the middle of the night, I got up and took a "header" across the bedroom and into the bathroom, knocking over everything in my path, before crashing into the bathtub. I was on a twenty four hour dose of chemotherapy that was packaged, complete with an electronic infusion pump. We new it was strong medicine, as we were sent home with a Hazardous Material Clean Up kit! For several days, I was off balance, as the left side of my body was temporarily neurologically "knocked out."

Another, more humorous time, Mary Lou was driving me home from the BMT center. We usually took the "scenic" route, off the major highway, with much less traffic. I think it was the only time I was nauseous on the way home, but I had to stop, and I had to stop right then! We pulled over, and I was obviously, and "forcefully displaying sickness," a local police officer stopped and started telling me I should have waited for the wider part of the road, about a mile further. An additional mile further was a mile too far, as there was no time! I appreciated the officer's concern for safety; however, I had no control over my nausea!

In general, a successful transplant requires the patient be healthy enough to undergo the demanding transplant process. Age, general physical condition, the patient's diagnosis and the stage of the disease are all considered by the transplant team when determining whether a person should undergo a transplant. I felt that I was in pretty decent physical conditioning, despite going through chemotherapy the year before.

Prior to my bone marrow transplant, several tests were carried out to ensure that I was physically capable of undergoing a transplant. For all BMT cases, tests of the patient's heart, lung, kidney and other vital organ functions are used to develop a patient "baseline" against which post-transplant tests can be compared, to determine if any body functions have been impaired. My physician and the BMT team thought I was in great condition and said they did not think the usual statistics would apply to me. It certainly was not a "cake walk," but I am sure it would have been much tougher without my principles of living a healthy life.

A bone marrow transplant requires an expert medical team—doctors, nurses, and other support staff—who can promptly recognize problems and emerging side effects, and know how to react swiftly and correctly if problems do arise. I cannot say enough about the transplant team at Rocky Mountain Blood and Marrow Transplant Practice, from the first encounter at the center's "front desk" to the contacts with my transplant physician "in-charge." It is impossible to single out good people—they were all that good! The same is true of the hospital BMT unit. Again, I cannot single out the great persons, as they were all top, caring professionals.

The Bone Marrow Harvest

The bone marrow harvest was a fairly simple procedure. Prior to harvesting, a small flexible "tube" or catheter (sometimes called a "Hickman®" or central venous line) was inserted into a large vein in my chest just above my heart.

I thought the PIC line was all I needed. However, since stem cells are relatively large, and the volume of blood that would be circulating through the tube required a bigger lumen (diameter), the "Hickman®" was added. The procedure consisted of a few days of a "couple" hour procedures in which my blood was continually pumped out through the central line, into a filtering machine to separate out and collect the stem cells, and return the remaining blood products back into my body. This central line, in addition would be useful later for the return of my stem cells, and also, like the PIC lines, enable the BMT medical staff to administer drugs and blood products to me easily, and to withdraw the hundreds of blood samples required during the course of treatment without inserting needles into my arms or hands.

The Preparative Regimen

Once, I had undergone "at home" chemotherapy, and the process of collecting my own donor cells, I was ready for my hospital visit. I packed the "best of my Aloha Hawaiian shirt collection, my Hawaiian CDs, my computer, and jokingly told my friends and family that I was going to an "extreme spa in Hawaii." I checked in, on my birthday, for a four week stay. I was admitted to the bone marrow transplant unit and within the first hour, I was undergoing the first of several days of high dose chemotherapy that would destroy my bone marrow and cancerous cells which would make room for the new bone marrow (my previously collected bone marrow that was frozen).

This is called the conditioning or preparative regimen. The exact regimen of chemotherapy and/or radiation varies according to the disease being treated and the "protocol" or preferred treatment plan of the facility where the BMT is being performed. I actually had a unique treatment plan that required an IRB (Investigational Review Board) approval and sign off.

The dosage of chemotherapy during conditioning is much stronger than dosages administered to me in my first chemo therapy sessions. It did not matter, as I was focused on "crossing the finish line," again, with my Ironman® medal, and my autographed jersey from Susan and the Northern California Chapter of Team In Training® group.

I had no obstacles to completing my treatment, only the "stepping stones" that I saw from the finish line. I celebrated every day, by rising, showering, turning on some Aloha music, and taking a "spin" on the stationary bike, that everyone assumed would be a "clothes rack." How wrong they were! All but one day, when I was too weak—blood levels too low, Dr's orders kept me off the bike. Otherwise, I was on it at least for a one hour ride, as I became weaker, I rode with no resistance, and extremely slow—but I rode!

Most days, I also walked up the hallway, past the "medical control desk," with my IV "tree" full of chemo and other IV bags of chemicals, attached by my PIC and Central lines. Since I was usually the only person out walking, I often passed the nurses and physicians who were silent, and looking up to see who would be walking around in the BMT unit, as the hallway was usually "stone silent" and any noise of a patient walking through was relatively rare. I knew the importance of exercise and I knew from the surprised looks on their faces as I walked by, as energetic and as often as I could, they would wonder how long I could keep up the pace. I was going to show up! I set up an expectation and I was going to meet it with my commitment! I was going to show my *"Unstoppable Attitude."*

Once, while I walked passed the nursing station, with my "tree" of IV bags in tow, I said *"I'm going to Starbucks®! Can I pick up anything for anyone?"* It took them a few seconds to consider the seriousness of my comment and, as I "ducked" into the patient's kitchenette, two of the nurses went running past to see if I had actually left the BMT unit. Of course, when they got to the end of the hallway, they realized that not even their "IronMan®" patient could move fast enough to escape!

A check of vital signs was performed by one of the nurses around the clock, every four hours. I also saw my transplant physician, or one of his partners once per day. I quickly realized how fast time went by, as I became weaker and slower!

Staying "well" is paramount in this process—the PIC and central lines must have entry sites that are infection free, food was prepared in a separate kitchen and brought to the room "gift wrapped" in clear plastic food wrap. If I had any fruit, such as an apple, it was washed, wrapped in food wrap, then I was to wash it once more in soap and water. The infection risk is so high in the BMT unit, as patients have no immune system. A germ that might give a normally healthy person a sniffle or two, could easily kill a BMT patient that does not have an immune system to fight it.

I recall once, a nurse was just leaving my room after taking my "vital" signs, just as a food tray was being brought in. As the food worker started for my door, the nurse immediately stuck her leg up across the doorway, preventing access. She noticed a piece of fruit that had not been wrapped. That is how careful they were—and vigilant!

Visitors to this unit had to "scrub up" each time they entered. I limited my visitors to one person, Mary Lou, who kept a set of comfortable pajamas in the room. She made them especially for this "extreme spa" adventure. In addition to "scrubbing up," she also took the precaution of changing out of her street clothes into her "visiting jams," even further reducing the chance of outside infections. "Germ free" was not an obstacle, I already planned ahead, as I saw it as a "stepping stone" to my success. I looked forward to Mary Lou's visits, but at the same time, I was also more and more aware of the toll it was taking on her. Being the loved ones of a cancer patient, I think, is tougher than being the patient.

Another event I enjoyed and looked forward to was calling my sister Sue, many nights after my 2:00am "vital signs check." Sue has always been a night person, and would just be getting home from work. For this reason, I was able to speak with her more than I have in years, as I am a day person!

It may sound strange, but it is true—while I love the sun and have fairly dark skin, my twin sister has dangerously fair skin, is allergic to the sun, and developed into a night person out of necessity. The times when we do get together, we compromise. I sit out in the sun, and we chat through a screen door, were she sits inside, in the shade. If you have the experience of going to confession, in the Catholic Church, you will appreciate the humor of that scene!

I also had my daily *"Unstoppable Attitude"* calls, from and to Kelly and Greg, when I would always get that "my world is a perfect place" feeling.

The Transplant Process

Time Line: 2001: February, March, April, May, June, July, August, September, October, November, December
Time Line: 2002: January, February, March, April, May, June, July, August, September, October, November, December
Time Line: 2003: January, February, March, April, May, June, July, August, September, October, November, December
Time Line: 2004: January, February, March, April

Exactly one week after the heavy doses of chemotherapy, I had my transplant. It was almost a serene spa treatment. I was ready, wearing my autograph yellow bicycle jersey from Susan and the Northern California Chapter of Team In Training®, and my Ironman® medal, again taken out of "retirement." My stem cells had been frozen, from my bone marrow, since harvesting, and were now being thawed to the right temperature.

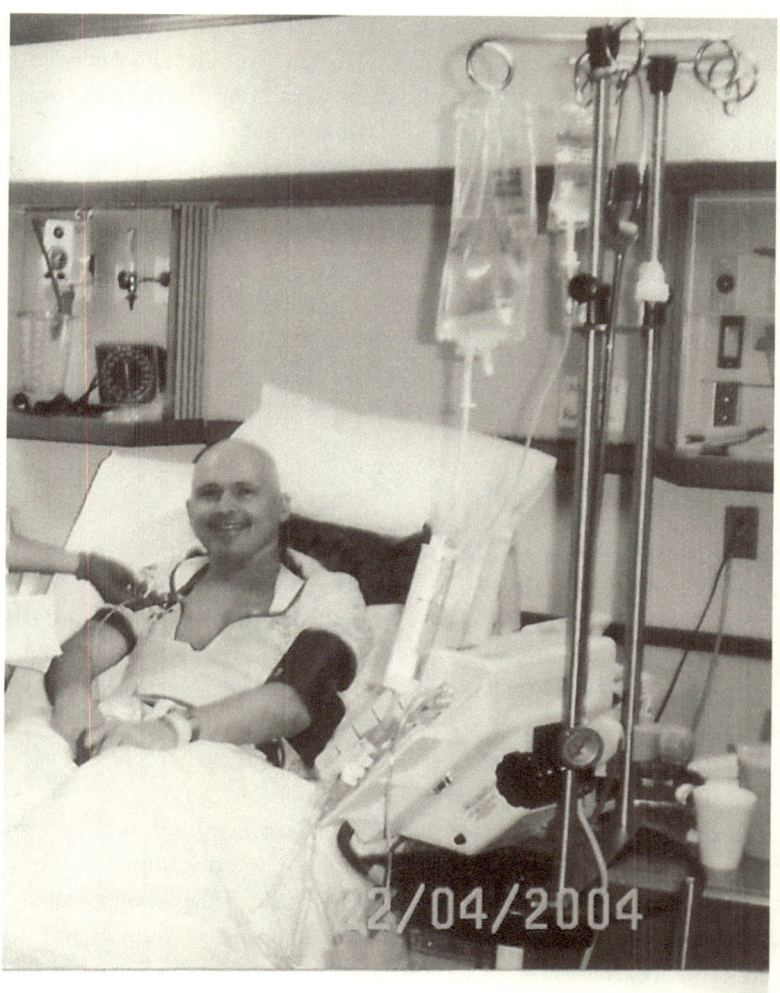

The Transplant Process

The entire transplantation was done in my room, and other than that, it is much the same as any blood product is given. The transplant is not a surgical procedure, nor painful experience. In fact, I found it a bit surreal. At the moment when the first of many IV bags was starting to be administered, Israel "Iz" Kamakawiwo'ole's rendition of "Somewhere Over The Rainbow," started playing on the CD player. I and the nurses were all silently "stunned" by the appropriateness of that song. Patients are checked frequently for signs of fever, chills, hives and chest pains while the bone marrow is being infused. If I was looking for a grand finale, this was not it, as this "race" was not over. The transplant, itself, was an easy and pleasant "stepping stone" towards the finish line.

That evening, I noticed a smell that I thought was a "dumpster fire" outside. I called for the nurse, who checked out the window for me and assured me there was no fire. The next morning, I could still smell a "smoldering dumpster" and expressed concern—I was finally "kindly made aware" that transplant patients often give off a "garlic" smell that comes from the frozen bone marrow preservative. In my case, as it was gently put, I smelled like a "smoldering dumpster" that people noticed as soon as they were in the BMT unit!

My Engraftment

The slightly less than two weeks, immediately following transplantation, were the most critical. The high-dose chemotherapy I had been given during conditioning was, as expected, still putting my immune system totally out of commission. In addition, while I was not receiving the high dose chemotherapy drugs, I was still going to be weakened further with side effects.

As I waited for the transplanted bone marrow to migrate to the cavities of the large bones, and "engraft," and begin producing normal blood cells, I was more and more very susceptible to infection and excessive bleeding. In fact, the bleeding and requirement of a transfusion of platelets is why my physician "benched" me one day from my "spin" on the bike. While the actual transplant was over, my IV "tree" had even more bags of chemicals emptying into my PIC and Central lines. In addition to the platelet transfusion, I also had several antibiotics to prevent and fight infection.

Extraordinary precautions were now taken to minimize my exposure to viruses and bacteria. The physicians and nurses now, even more carefully, routinely washed their hands with antiseptic soap, right outside my door, and wore clean protective gowns, gloves and often masks while in my room. Blood samples were taken daily to determine whether or not engraftment had occurred and to monitor organ function. When my transplanted bone marrow began to engraft and started to produce normal blood cells, I was gradually taken off the antibiotics. I left the hospital after a three week stay, one week earlier than planned.

I Leave The Hospital

Time Line: 2001: February, March, April, May, June, July, August, September, October, November, December
Time Line: 2002: January, February, March, April, May, June, July, August, September, October, November, December
Time Line: 2003: January, February, March, April, May, June, July, August, September, October, November, December
Time Line: 2004: January, February, March, April, May

My recovery continued at home. It had now been about three years since I first sought medical help for my "sore hip". We were still in the "race," keeping our home as clean as possible, and going through the "heparin flushing" process of the PIC and Central lines. I was also giving myself daily injections, in my belly, of a cell growth stimulant. I had daily appointments with my team at the BMT center, which turned into twice a week, then once a week. I did not know it, but one of my worse experiences was yet to come. My PIC line was removed, and was a simple procedure. An interventional radiologist simply pulled it out of my arm.

When my own immune system was strong enough, I went back to the hospital to have my central line removed. This required minor surgery—at most a local anesthetic would be used. When I was called in, the interventional radiologists met me and explained that he did not usually work at this hospital and was just "filling in" for someone.

He asked: *"How long has your central line been in?"*

I replied: *"Only about eight weeks."*

Dr: *"This will be easy. Sometimes, if the line has been in for a few months, it will become part of the scar tissue that develops, and requires some sedation. When it's only been in a few weeks, it is simply a local anesthetic and a tug."*

He turned towards the one nurse that was present and said: *"this will be simple—go ahead and take your lunch break."*

The tugging, despite the "local anesthetic," was painful, and he started working with the scalpel. He sensed my heart rate and temperature going up, as I sensed his intensity level going up. As he worked deeper and deeper, I was clenching my teeth tighter and tighter as he got closer and closer to see what he was doing.

As he approached with his face about a six inch distance from my chest he said those dreaded words: *"Oh-Oh."*

Before I could focus on an outcome and plan my "stepping stones," I already had taken on a "muscle through this attitude."

Dr: *"I'm sorry, I started this ... I need to finish—I am so sorry,..... .this thing looks like it has been in for years. I'll keep squirting in the Lidocaine ...—just let me know when you need it—I don't have help now ... I don't know where other supplies are that I can reach quickly..... . I am so sorry!"*

It seemed like an eternity to get the line released from my body and pulled out. I went out into the waiting area, where Mary Lou was waiting. She had a shocked look on her face when she saw me, as I was completely drenched with perspiration, and shaking with physical stress. It was actually the worse pain I experienced through all of my entire cancer treatments. I quickly put it behind me, and I do not blame the physician. It was a bad experience for him, as well, and he was "up front" enough to admit the mistake. His mistake was that he went by how I looked, and that the "normal" patient's central line should be an easy removal process. Thankfully, I know there are future patients that will benefit from this awful experience.

Time Line: 2001: February, March, April, May, June, July, August, September, October, November, December
Time Line: 2002: January, February, March, April, May, June, July, August, September, October, November, December
Time Line: 2003: January, February, March, April, May, June, July, August, September, October, November, December
Time Line: 2004: January, February, March, April, May, June, July

I started a 25 day course of radiation treatment in which the old "sweet spot" was targeted from my back as well as my front. Radiation was the simple part of my entire "race," and, by now, I drove myself to most treatments. Every treatment was identical, and it only took a few treatments before it became a routine and I did not need to be prompted to: *"unbuckle your belt, unzip your pants, and roll down your waist band."* In fact, it became such a routine that when I was finally well enough to go through airport security for the first time after my treatments, and I was prompted to: *"take your shoes and belt off and put them on the conveyor."* I, in fact, unbuckled my belt, unzipped my pants, and started to roll my waist band before I heard a security guard yell *"stop!—What are you doing?"*

**Time Line**: 2001: February, March, April, May, June, July, August, September, October, November, December
**Time Line**: 2002: January, February, March, April, May, June, July, August, September, October, November, December
**Time Line**: 2003: January, February, March, April, May, June, July, August, September, October, November, December
**Time Line**: 2004: January, February, March, April, May, June, July

I was anxious to return to work. I walked into corporate headquarters, unannounced, just across the street from the division I ran before I left. I seemed to alarm people and realized "something was up" other than my bald head. The assistant to the CEO asked if I had been to my office yet and I replied that I thought I should "check in" first. She seemed very relieved of this.

I met with the CEO and he explained that the success I had achieved with my division had resulted in a necessity to move someone into my spot. He asked if I would take over another division that was struggling, and confidentially and carefully implied that the parent company was selling off the entire organization. So, I agreed and started to look elsewhere, but not before I began to train the great young people of this new group, in the principles of "*Unstoppable Attitude.*"

I am now a full time "coach," teaching "responsible" marketing courses to very inspiring future "authentic leaders" at the University of Colorado at Denver and Health Science center. I approach every class as a motivational and training meeting, and it is wonderfully inspiring, rewarding, and at times, outrageously exhausting in such a good way. When I see the many wonderful young people leave my classes with "*Unstoppable Attitude,*" all is right with the world!

7

The Ten Principles Of "Unstoppable Attitude"

Principle 1: Be Inspired

The sources of inspiration are endless. The "key" is simple—just be open to inspiration. My children inspire me greatly! My co-workers who really "show up" in life have inspired me, and my current students and colleagues at the University of Colorado at Denver School of Business greatly inspire me. Inspiration gives you energy from other sources than only your own.

Principle 2: Mentally Place Yourself At The Finish Line

Focus is so important. I need the focus of a "finish line," so that I can mentally turn around and mentally change those "obstacles" into "stepping stones." Once you can mentally place yourself at the "finish line," every crossing of a "stepping stone" becomes a celebration. Thus, *celebrate your goals before you achieve them.*

Principle 3: Live Healthy, Exercise, Eat Well

Interestingly, I often meet a skeptic that says something like *"all the effort you have put into exercise, eating the right foods, etc., sure hasn't paid off for you!"* I am, even more convinced now, than ever before. Bad "stuff," beyond peoples' control does, indeed, happen. Had I not been in good shape I would not have had such a comparatively "easy" time of the whole cancer treatment process. Don't get me wrong—this was tough. However, people who had the toughest time seemed to have the least lifetime fitness preparation for the "race of their life."

Principle 4: Be An Involved Life Learner

Once you have a focus on what you are going to accomplish, acquire as much knowledge as possible. I cannot say I became an expert on cancer, but I became as knowledgeable as I could. I continually wondered how cancer patients and their families made it through the process without a good understanding of what they were going through.

Principle 5: Find A Coach

From the sports world, I knew the importance of a good coach. From the business world I also knew the importance of a good coach. From the cancer world, I know a good coach is someone who has good advice from a sound base of knowledge and when in doubt, does not hesitate to seek good advice from other good coaches, and takes initiative to communicate well with me. A good coach exhibits and lives what they want me to believe in. My great coach, Dr Carol, has "*Unstoppable Attitude*" and lives an authentic healthy life.

Principle 6: Be A Coach

I believe I became more knowledgeable about what motivates people, what inspires them and what makes "*Authentic Leadership*" such an imperative, easily attained, yet so scarce a commodity. We need more inspiring coaches, in all walks of life.

Principle 7: Do Not Ask Why Me?—Ask Why Not Me?

Why not me?—I can do this! (and so can you!)

Principle 8: Inspire Others To, In Turn, Inspire Others

To really appreciate that "all is right with the world" feeling, go beyond inspiring someone. Make sure part of the inspiration is "passed on." When it starts to come back automatically, you receive "those moments".

Principle 9: Surround Yourself With Positive Supporting People

Sports and business taught me the value of positive people on my teams. Cancer taught me it is a necessity that is priceless. It is a rough road to go alone, and I cannot imagine success at focusing on crossing "my finish lines" without my supportive "teams"

Principle 10: Make Your Miles Quality Miles

Sports and business also taught me the value of "going the distance." Cancer taught me the value of "quality" miles. I could have been just treated for a bone disease or cancer and "survived." In fact, I believe that no one merely "survives" cancer—they work at it. Mary Lou, in fact, uses the phrase "Cancer Thrivers". I choose to adopt my "Unstoppable Attitude" and was one of the fortunate people that triumphed! I was not the only one running "quality miles". Dr. Carol, my endocrinologist "ran quality miles" in my race, "promoted" me to other physicians for their opinions, and carried my charts and scans to several medical meetings—she persisted, with *quality*, for the entire distance.

I also know, without a doubt, that the most effective way to move forward, with "quality miles" towards *"Unstoppable Attitude"* is not to dwell in the past. **Nothing holds people from forward progress more that anger about what was or what was not done in the past**. This can be a huge impasse to our *"Unstoppable Attitude."* There is, as I have said before, just a "plain and simple" time to energize all our resources to move ahead.

8

Just A Few Of My Heartfelt Acknowledgements

I cannot end my story with a simple page of acknowledgements. The people I acknowledge deserve, at the very least, an entire chapter!

To all cancer patients, their spouses, partners, and loved ones that have run their "races" before me, particularly to those, despite their valiant efforts, were not able to cross the "survival finish line" of cancer. You and your very loved and missed cancer hero's are the true champions of this amazing process. It is your hard work, dedication, and ultimate sacrifices that have paved the way for my self and thousands of others to cross the cancer "survival finish line".

Of course, Kelly and Greg, you both inspire me. You are solid citizens of the world, and, although you have established your homes on each coast, you so very, very often give me that "all is right with the world" feeling. You have chosen partners and positive support teams around you. You inspire others, you are life long learners, and you live healthy lives. The Boston, New York, Chicago, and San Francisco marathons, as well as the several Ironman® and Danskin® triathlons you have challenged, and the whole world, are all better because of your "quality miles," "authentic leadership," and *"Unstoppable Attitudes."*

My sister Sue and her husband Tom. The BMT process gave me an opportunity to get to know my favorite "night" person. Their overwhelming desire to make things easy or better, despite living seven hundred miles away was truly appreciated. Sue became the "point person" for my side of the family and relayed the many prayers and positive thoughts from my brothers and their wives.

Mary Lou's family, especially her sister Nancy and her mom, Julia, sent their prayers and well wishes, as did Michael and Mila. Julia's battle with her own cancer, during my final treatments did not slow down the energy she sent my way!

I have been a beneficiary of past research the Leukemia & Lymphoma Society's Team In Training® efforts have supported. Since 1988, more than 295,000 volunteer participants have helped raise more than $660 million for cancer, much going directly to funding cancer research grants. I have also personally benefited with an "Unstoppable Attitude" boost from my friend Susan and her Northern California Chapter, whose yellow jersey—signed by each member of her team—I wore across each "finish line" of my two cancer victories! Susan is now coaching a team, raising further awareness and funds for cancer research. I and Mary Lou have recently joined The Rocky Mountain Chapter of Team In Training®.

I acknowledge my admiration for patients that have, through their bravery in agreeing to experimental clinical trials for the development of new therapies, immeasurably added to my chance of success and the success of thousands of others. It is because of you that my cancer success and those of countless others has been possible. Your bravery to step into somewhat "unknown" therapies cannot be acknowledged enough!

I refer to Dr. Carol as my "coach." I could write paragraphs about her *"Unstoppable Attitude,"* her "authentic leadership," her professionalism, her persistence, etc. I am sure she received much criticism from cancer experts, being told she was wrong about my case. As a physician, she distinguished herself by looking at me as more than a patient with laboratory values and CT scans. She questioned my healthy appearance, asked other questions, sought out information from other experts, and continually coached me on what to do next. Before anyone else, she knew I did not "fit" the statistical norms for patients, and therefore questioned the lab and test results. What makes her a true "standout" is that she treats all her patients this way. I will sum it up by simply stating what has become obvious to me: Without her, I would not be here!

As a great healing environment during my first cancer Ironman®, Westminster Front Range Community College Colleagues and students provided a unique experience. I was not part of the educational process, as I worked for the Governor's Office of Economic Development and my office just "happened" to be there. However, I greatly benefited from that environment. Linda, my "point person" at the college, while being exceptionally helpful with my work was also unique with her compassionate humor, and Christine, who lost her husband to cancer only a few months prior to my diagnosis, and the many other folks that joined me for a walk up and down that long hallway a couple of times a day—all had such positive energy they passed on to me!

The great folks at Proligo®, "the DNA factory" (no longer in existence), particular Paula, the director of sales, whom I spoke with often during the BMT process. She is an "authentic leader with *"Unstoppable Attitude"* that really carried the division during my BMT. Paula's Mom, whom I have not met, always sent her well wishes to me, through Paula, and made sure I knew she was praying for me. Jennifer, one of two laboratory and production managers and I, used to have our daily production meeting while walking a couple of miles, during lunch. She told me she wanted some exercise, and I was secretly training for my BMT. In addition, her previous position was as a transplant nurse with a BMT unit. As the possibility of a BMT was becoming more evident, she unknowingly helped with my "pre" BMT education process. Joey, a corporate VP who was instrumental in hiring me for my "Unstoppable Attitude", was very perceptive (to recognize "Unstoppable Attitude," one must have it themselves—and she does!). She would notice me, walking across the street, from my building, to the corporate offices, and suspected a second bout of cancer, several weeks before my oncologist confirmed it!

Sam, my good friend is not mentioned in my notes yet, he was always there and was a very important and consistent member of my support team, through both cancer Ironman® races. Sam had an uncanny ability to "show up," at just the right times, with his almost weekly appearance, or by telephone and ask: "am I catching you at an O.K. time?" Sam also is an "authentic leader" with *"Unstoppable Attitude"* and is a master of "compassion with a sense of humor." Sam, you always show up at an O.K. time! Sam is now a winner of his own "Cancer Race."

As I stated before, Rocky Mountain Blood and Marrow Transplant Practice was of the highest professional caliber. For me, the people at this center were a very "confidence building" group. RMBMT Center was truly the professional, supportive team that surrounded me and my primary care provider, Mary Lou. I cannot single out a single person, nor would anyone there want me to single out anyone as "particularly great"—They were all particularly great!

The same is true for the BMT unit at Presbyterian St. Luke's Medical Center in Denver. The facilities and professional people were compassionate "confidence builders." They too, were all particularly great.

I warmly acknowledge the University of Colorado at Denver and Health Science center School of Business. Since I was an adjunct professor of marketing, I taught one evening class per semester in the MBA program. I therefore saw students, but rarely saw any colleagues, unless I was early enough to stop by the main office. On those rare occasions, I would stop by to see Cliff. Since he saw me so infrequently, during my first "race" against cancer, I always felt I needed to re-introduce myself, as my looks kept changing so much. When he realized it was me, he always had such an outpouring of positive energy. I "just got" that he was proud I was teaching a class at the University and proud I was taking care of my "cancer business" in such a positive manner. Marti was the same way. I so infrequently saw her, but when I did, she made certain I was O.K. Renee always made sure I knew of her prayers and support. Of course, the graduate MBA marketing class, that witnessed my first "race" was very inspiring, often in such simple ways. Prior to the start of class, as I was sanitizing the desk and equipment, they would "check out" how my looks had changed since the prior week. A simple "thumbs up" from many of them assured me of my "quality miles" in that "race." The most inspiring event was the evening of the last class, in which a student told me that his wife was surprised that he never missed one of my classes. He said he liked the class, but he would not dare miss a class, knowing I was going to be there! He said he was truly inspired to "show up."

Now that I am a full time faculty member at the University of Colorado at Denver and Health Science Center, I receive outstanding support often, from the many faculty and administration people in the School of Business. It is, like Rocky Mountain Blood and Bone Marrow Transplant Cancer, a place that is impossible to single out great people—as they all are!

Lance Armstrong is someone I find tremendously inspiring. So much has been written about him, his success over cancer, and his outstanding cycling accomplishments inspired me to use one of his quotes as part of my Email signature: *"I show up prepared, I show up motivated and I show up because I love it and respect it and I want to do well."*

I know there are many people who prayed for me and had well wishes that were "silent". They either did not want to bother me, or they did not know how to speak their minds to me, directly. I want you to know how much I received from you!

Crossing the "finish line" of writing this book, I finally, but not lastly in importance, acknowledge the unsung heroes—the people who show the most bravery and compassion, and those who suffer far, far more than cancer patients. These folks are the spouses, partners, and loved ones of cancer patients. In acknowledging my wife, Mary Lou, I also acknowledge all of the others. I not only witnessed the experience of Mary Lou, albeit through my mental "chemo fog." I spoke to a number of patients' partners to "solidly come to my place" of compassion, respect, and admiration for these beautiful folks.

Cancer is particularly a tough ordeal on partners and loved ones. They desperately want and need to be fighting "in the race." Most of the time, however, they cannot, and when they can, they feel it is never enough. They are forced into a "limbo" state. They can only watch as they can try to carry on with their jobs, constantly apologizing for missing meetings, not focusing, leaving work early, etc. It was only in the BMT process that Mary Lou felt she became a "true" team member, when she was assigned the responsibility of "flushing" out my lines. Even with a chance to be physically involved with actual treatment, she was constantly aware that a "mistake" could result in an infection, and subsequently her partner's life! I can only imagine that kind of pressure.

The cancer patients' partners witness the "worst of the worse" being inflicted on "the" someone they love. In return, they finish many days of chauffeuring their partner to and from medical centers, catching up on their own jobs, then facing a growing pile of clinic and insurance correspondence that even an insurance agent would find insurmountable. In many cases the job of "defensive point person" is delegated to the cancer patients' partners. People call constantly to check on the patients' status, intensions good—asking "when can we visit," "why can't we visit," "why can't we send flowers," (risk of fungi or germ infections) and repeat these inquires, often—too often, without asking; "so tell me, "patients' partner," how are *you* doing."

The special champions are those that, despite their valiant efforts, did not see their loved ones cross the cancer survival "finish line."

To all of these wonderful, lovely, folks, particularly my wife, Mary Lou:

You are the true champions of this whole process. It is you whom I love, and for you whom the memories of my "first," "second" and "third" Ironman® events are written for!

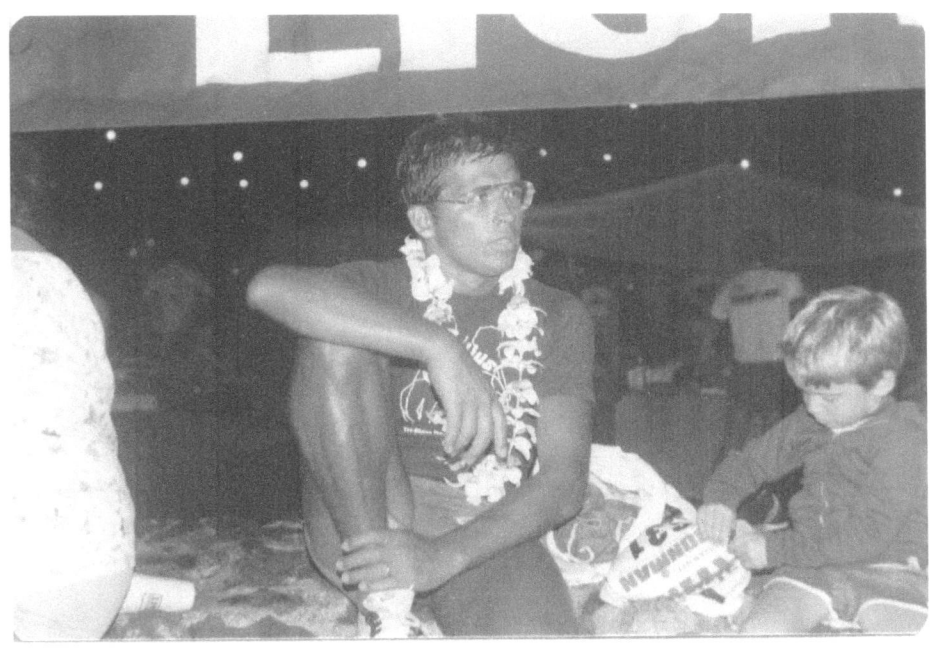

Dad and Greg After Dad's 1982 Ironman World Championship

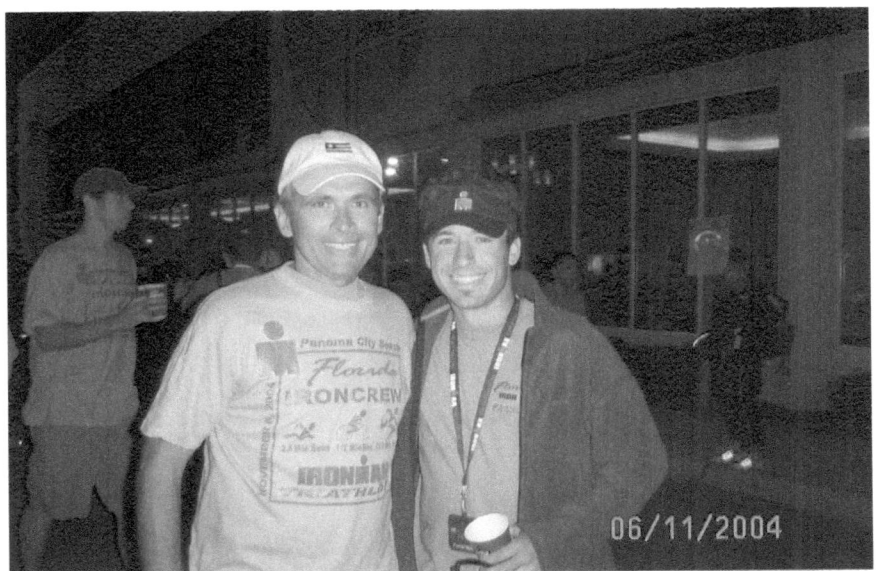

Dad and Greg after Greg's 2004 Ironman® Panama City Triathlon

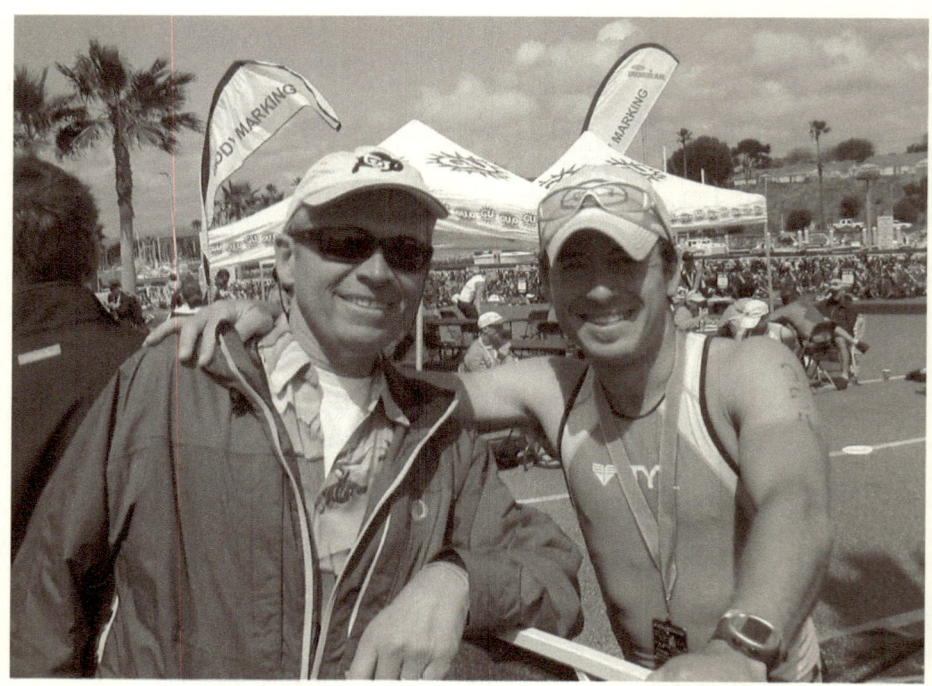

Dad and Greg at Greg's Ironman® Ocean City Triathlon 2005

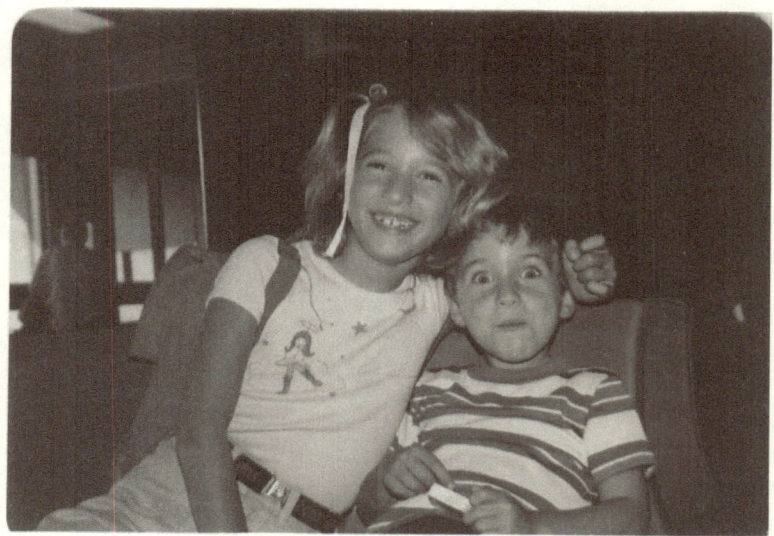

Kelly and Greg at Dad's 1982 Ironman® World Championship event

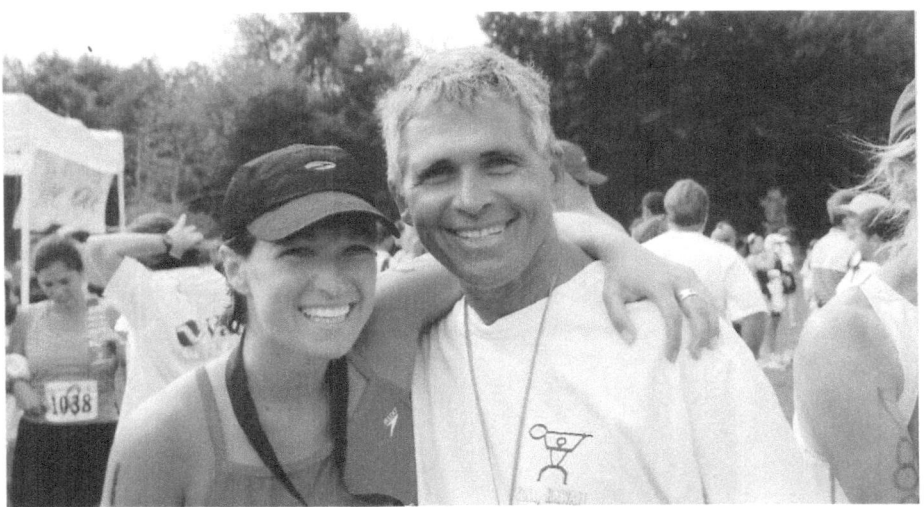

Dad and Kelly after one of her Danskin® Triathlons in 2004

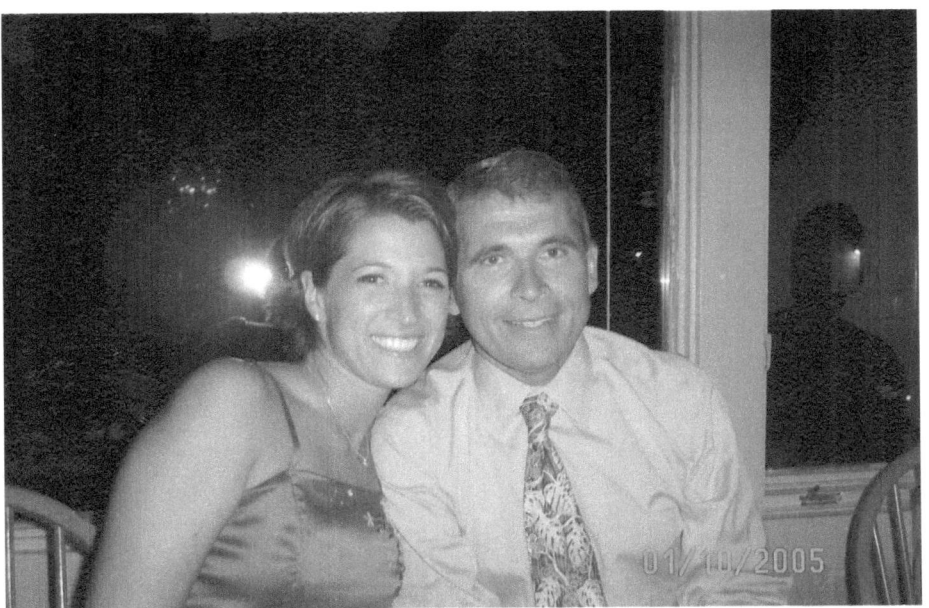

Dad and Kelly after Kelly's 2005 Wedding!

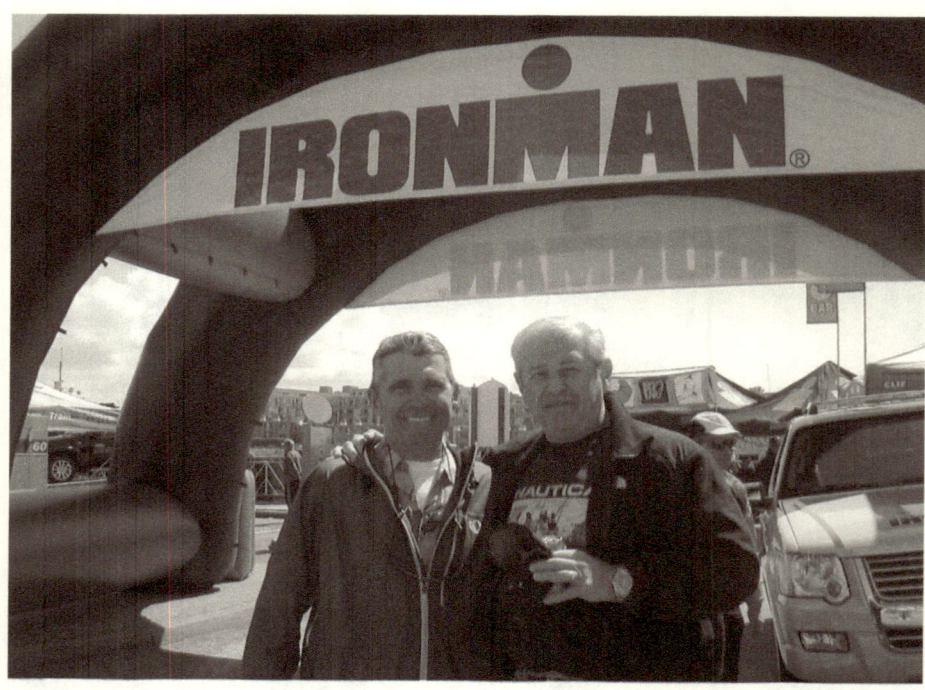

At Greg's Ironman® Ocean City Triathlon, with my friend, Sam—now a winner over his own Cancer Championship!

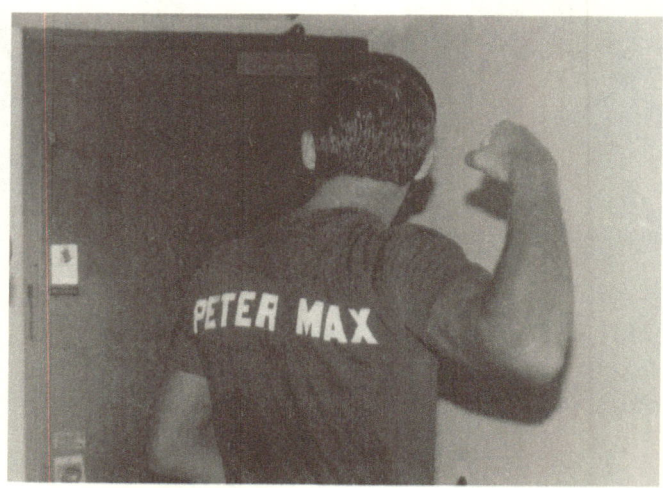

Before 1982 Ironman® displaying "Unstoppable Attitude", and how I start each and every challenge!

About the Author

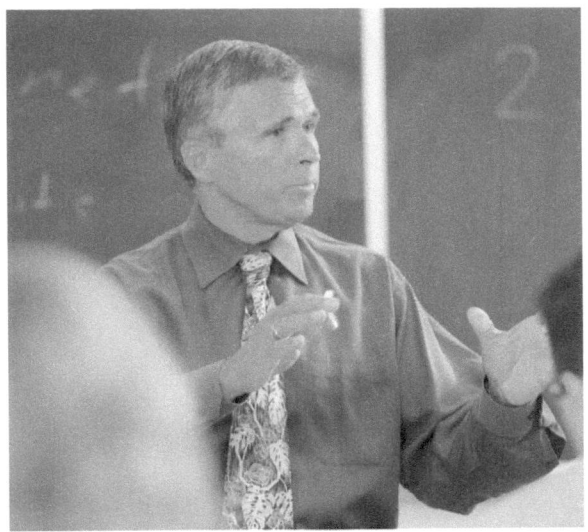

PeterMax Miller is available for motivational speaking and training. His "coaching" focus is organizational marketing and sales groups, as well as oncology support groups including patient support (families, loved ones) and support office staff, nurses, and physicians.

For information: www.UnstoppableAttitude.com

978-0-595-49224-4
0-595-49224-X